I0112548

WHY BLACK PEOPLE DIE SOONER

Why Black People Die Sooner

WHAT MEDICINE GETS WRONG ABOUT
RACE AND HOW TO FIX IT

Joseph L. Graves Jr.

Columbia University Press
New York

Columbia University Press
Publishers Since 1893
New York   Chichester, West Sussex
cup.columbia.edu

Cataloging-in-Publication Data available from the Library of Congress.
ISBN 9780231217965 (hardback)
ISBN 9780231561990 (ebook)

LCCN 2025010386

Printed in the United States of America

Cover design: Julia Kushnirsky
Cover image: Shutterstock

GPSR Authorized Representative: Easy Access System Europe,
Mustamäe tee 50, 10621 Tallinn, Estonia, gpsr.requests@easproject.com

For Beth . . . Rest in peace and power

CONTENTS

PREFACE

This psalm is attributed to Moses. Moses is one of the most important
prophets of Judaism, Christianity, and Islam. Religious texts say that he was
born under the reign of a pharaoh who had enslaved the children of Israel
sometime in the thirteenth century BCE. Archaeologists view Moses as a
legendary figure, not a real person. The reality of the prophet makes no
difference to the arguments I am about to make in this text. However, it is
interesting to note that Moses felt that the lifespan of the people of his time
(including those living under the yoke of slavery) was about seventy years
and that the strongest of them made it to eighty years.

This becomes more interesting in the context of the environment in which
these people labored. They subsisted on an agricultural diet, undoubtedly
without any food in excess of their daily needs. The enslaved may have
been driven by the lash and given little rest in subtropical temperatures.
They would have been exposed to viral, bacterial, malarial, and helminth
infections. Thus, while this psalm is poetic, I doubt its accuracy. We have no
way to validate its claims since the archaeological finds of human remains
from this region and time period are generally limited to the masters, not
their slaves.

However, we do know about the lifespans of human beings under chattel
slavery in the Americas and the current-day lifespans of their descendants.
The mean lifespan of enslaved people varied by state but never reached
seventy years. In the 1890s, African Americans were dying at rates that

prompted some scholars to propose that the "race" might be extinct by the turn of the century. Of course, this didn't happen, and the lifespans of all Americans gradually increased over the twentieth century—but with a persistent gap between European and African Americans. The mean lifespan of African Americans exceeded seventy years by the beginning of the twenty-first century. From 2006 to 2019, the mean life expectancy from birth ranged from seventy-two to seventy-five years for African Americans and was over seventy-eight years for European Americans.

This book examines why there has been a consistent difference in lifespan between African and European Americans and the role that our society, and the medical profession in particular, has played in perpetuating this gap. I will argue that the origin of modern medicine within the confines of false racial beliefs negatively influenced its practice and that such beliefs persist in the twenty-first century. Indeed, it might shock you to know that nineteenth-century racial thinking still plays a role in the training of physicians. These misconceptions, in combination with physicians' implicit racial biases, inherited from a society still driven by structural racism, continue to cause harm to African Americans and other racially subordinated people.

The simple explanation for the difference in lifespan between African and European Americans is genetic differences between these groups. Western racial science began with the belief that Africans were inferior to Europeans in virtually every biological and cultural trait. This belief has been shown to be patently false, but in this book, I will not take a deep dive into topics such as the nature of human biological differentiation or the differences between biological and social conceptions of race. The reader who wishes more background on these subjects is directed to my previous works.[1] That said, I will provide sufficient background for the reader to understand how human biological variation operates in the context of the diseases and medical procedures discussed.

Throughout this work, I shall try to consistently describe human biological ancestry using geographical terms such as *African American, Asian American,* and *European American.* Since all socially defined racial terms are imprecise, it really doesn't matter which scheme you choose to discuss racialized groups, but it does matter that you explain to the reader which scheme you are using and why that scheme is best for the topic under discussion. When I cite material from the existing biomedical literature, I use the terms deployed by the authors of the literature in question. The terms

Black and *white* are often encountered in the medical literature. When you see these terms in the text, they refer to people whose primary ancestry is from Africa or Europe, respectively. The ancestry profile of Black people varies dramatically by geographic region. Africans are not one population. Structure-type genetic analysis indicates that there are at least four major population groups of Indigenous Africans (see chapters 8 and 9). The majority of Africans enslaved in the Western Hemisphere had their origins in West or Central Africa. Because of the various pattens of slavery in the West, Blacks have various amounts of African, European, and Native American ancestry. Because of the social norms of colonialism and slavery, the term *white* refers to people who are of primarily European ancestry. Finally, when I refer to the historical literature, I will use the terms used by the authors of those works. The terms used to describe human groups have changed over time. Some may be offensive to readers, but I think it is important to use them in their historical and cultural context to help us better understand how racism operated in the time periods discussed.

Thus, the purpose of *Why Black People Die Sooner* is to explain why modern medicine still operates under false conceptions of race, how those false conceptions cause harm to patients, and how we can change things.

WHY BLACK PEOPLE DIE SOONER

INTRODUCTION

Medicine Has Always Gotten Race Wrong

But what the small-pox spar's . . . the flux swept off. . . . after all our pains and care
to give them their messes in due order and season, keeping their lodgings as clean
and sweet as possible, and enduring so much misery and stench so long among a
parcel of creatures nastier than swine; and after all our expectations to be defeated
by their mortality.

CAPTAIN THOMAS PHILLIPS, COMPLAINING ABOUT THE HIGH
MORTALITY RATE ON HIS SLAVE SHIP, THE *HANNIBAL*, 1693

Built in London, the slave ship *Hannibal* has gone down in history for
its disastrous voyage carrying enslaved people from the African port of
modern-day Benin to Barbados between 1693 and 1695. The ship, 25 feet
wide and 100 feet long, was designed to carry 450 passengers on what was
known as the "Middle Passage" of the Atlantic slave trade. But its captain
was so eager to maximize the return on his investment that he decided to
pack 700 men, women, and children into the ship's bottom decks, almost
twice its capacity. For the African prisoners, chained together in "slave
racks" where they could not fully sit up, the two-month voyage across the
Atlantic was a living hell. Some even jumped off the ship to their death. In
all, 328 enslaved people—almost half (47 percent)—died before reaching
Barbados, mostly from "white flux" (dysentery) and smallpox.

There was, unfortunately, nothing special about the *Hannibal*. Conditions on ships in the slave triangle were universally horrendous. Disease
was rampant: from diarrhea to dysentery, malaria, smallpox, yellow fever,
measles, typhoid, hookworm, tapeworm, trypanosomiasis, syphilis, leprosy,
and elephantiasis. Women were raped repeatedly. Enslaved people suffered
from friction sores, ulcers, wounds, and injuries from accidents, fights, and
whippings. The average mortality rate for enslaved people aboard ships in
the British slave trade was 17 percent.[1]

When British slave traders realized that the bad conditions on the ships
were costing them money, they hired physicians to sail the Middle Passage

to keep their cargo alive. Far from an act of humanity, however, this was considered simply a cost of business. It was also a lucrative trade for physicians, who were generally paid for each enslaved person they managed to keep alive over the voyage. One of the most famous slave ship doctors was the eighteenth-century naval surgeon Alexander Falconbridge (1769–1792), who left an account of his efforts to keep slaves as healthy as possible during the long Middle Passage. He wrote that the conditions were so sickening that "it is not in the power of the human imagination to picture a situation more dreadful or disgusting."[2]

Falconbridge subsequently quit the slave ship trade and became an abolitionist, but he was an exception to the rule. Most involved in selling African slaves had no qualms about trading human lives or killing human beings. How? By convincing themselves that Africans were not actually human or that they were so genetically inferior that their deaths were somehow natural and unavoidable. Seventy-six years after the voyage of the *Hannibal*, Joseph Lewis, the personal physician to Dartmouth College's president, Eleazar Wheelock, became infamous for peeling the skin from a deceased enslaved man named Cato, boiling his body in a kettle to free the flesh from the bone, and using his skeleton for anatomical study. Cato's skin was then tanned and used to dress the doctor's instrument case.[3]

After losing control over their own bodies, enslaved Africans became material for the medical world to use to develop new techniques and further its understanding of anatomy. In fact, during the eighteenth century in Britain and beyond, the success of a medical college was tied directly to its ability to acquire bodies for anatomical dissection. As far as the colleges were concerned, African bodies were there for the taking. In 1762, the University of Pennsylvania hospital donated the body of a Negro who had died from suicide to the director of the university's anatomy course. In New York, King's College dug up cadavers from the Negroes Burying Ground (later named the African Burial Grounds) to use in teaching and experimentation. In 1773, the body of a Negro was used to produce the skeleton for anatomy lessons in Providence, Rhode Island.

THE NEGRO: "SOME OTHER KIND OF SPECIES"

While many people today consider the horrors of the slave trade and the use of African American bodies for medical experimentation remnants of a past that has been censured and corrected, the history of slavery shows that ideas don't die with the institutions that create them. Instead, they get updated to fit new contexts and institutions. In the case of slavery, Western medicine's first encounters with Africans took place aboard slave ships, embedding racist misconceptions in the foundation of American medicine. The idea that African bodies were not fully human, or that Africans were "some other kind of species," was established, updated, and integrated into new medical practices as they developed. The result is many racist assumptions that remain in medicine today. Structural racism killed Black people during slavery, Reconstruction, Jim Crow, and the civil rights era, and racist ideology continues to negatively affect how well Black Americans are diagnosed and the quality of the medical treatment they receive.

Racial misconceptions in medicine started with classifying physical differences as signs of inferiority. Throughout the eighteenth century, American physicians identified a host of biological, anatomical, and behavioral features that they believed proved that Negroes were inferior to whites of European ancestry. In 1798, the founding father and physician Benjamin Rush claimed that "blackness" was a form of leprosy that physicians might cure in the future.[4] In 1799, the physicians William H. Harvey and John Lindsey identified a disease they called "Cachexia Africana," which was characterized by people of African descent eating dirt in reaction to emotional distress and depression.[5] It turned out that this condition was not a pathology at all but rather a cultural practice in many tropical countries associated with treating iron deficiency.[6]

But by this time, nothing could contradict the narrative that portrayed the Negro as inherently defective. Over and over, throughout the centuries, conclusions about the state of Negroes' health were drawn to reinforce a desire to keep Blacks in a state of servitude. Southern physicians claimed that enslaved Africans were more physiologically suited to hard labor in the subtropical and tropical climates of the southernmost English colonies than were Europeans.[7] How surprising is that? Physicians on slave ships worked for slave sellers, and during the antebellum period (1832–1860), physicians in the United States made handsome incomes helping slave owners keep their slaves healthy enough to work. They would have gained nothing and lost much by challenging racist assumptions about Negroes.

The descendants of African slaves could not win against this circular racist reasoning. Even when physicians discussed the relative strengths of Black slaves, their observations became justifications for perpetuating slavery. The fact that darker skin provided greater protection from damaging ultraviolet rays than did fair skin was cited as proof that Negroes were designed by God to work in the sun. The plantation owner Philip Tidyman (1776–1850) argued that the nature of Africans' constitutions protected them from the dangers of hot climates and made them well suited to hard labor. The Louisiana physician Samuel Cartwright (1793–1863) claimed that African eyes were better suited to harsh sunlight—in the same way that orangutans' eyes were.

Conclusions like this flew in the face of abundant factual evidence to the contrary. Properly clothed and taking in adequate amounts of water and salt, poor people of European descent—most of whom were the descendants of indentured servants—also managed to work long hours in the subtropical sun. Yet to fend off moral objections to slavery altogether, highly respected nineteenth-century physicians argued that Negroes were a species of human distinct from Europeans. The physician and scientist Samuel Morton (1799–1851) used the notion of polygenism to this end. Polygenism, the idea of the separate creation of different human species, originated in the sixteenth century but did not become "scientifically" popular until the nineteenth century. Morton argued that contrary to "monogenism"—the belief that human races originated from a single pair of humans—various "races" of humanity were, in fact, different biological species. Naturally, Africans came out as the inferior race in this theory.[8] To support his argument, Morton amassed a collection of skulls from some one thousand individuals to study their cranial capacity. He concluded that the cranial volumes of so-called inferior species were less than those of Europeans.[9]

And then came Samuel Cartwright, an internationally recognized figure in medicine who was considered an expert on pneumonia, croup, fever, and cholera and who had received an award from Harvard University for his work on veins and absorption, as well as a medal from the Boston Medical Society for an essay on resuscitating drowning victims. Despite his impressive suite of accomplishments, Cartwright was perfectly comfortable using faulty racist logic in his attempt to scientifically prove the inferiority of the Negro. In his 1851 *Report on the Diseases and Physical Peculiarities of the Negro Race*, addressed to the Medical Association of Louisiana, he defined and documented "African" diseases, including drapetomania (an insane desire to run away), rascality (unruliness), and dysesthesia ethiopica (performing tasks in a haphazard manner).[10]

Cartwright's views were thoroughly in line with the racial thinking of most of his Southern physician colleagues at the time. After all, these physicians' skills were evaluated on the basis of how accurately they could judge the resale value of enslaved people. In this vein, Cartwright believed that he was helping physicians become fully aware of the "special diseases" to which the Negro was subject.[11] Yet modern medicine to this day has still not completely escaped the principles of racial difference that Cartwright established: his conception of racial difference was taught to tens of thousands of American medical students in the nineteenth century.

SLAVERY ENDED, BUT HEALTH DISPARITIES REMAINED

The Civil War demonstrated that racism outlives the institutions that create it. The war was a long, bitter struggle that ended slavery but did little to end racism. At its conclusion, formerly enslaved people—who had begun to escape in large numbers as early as 1862—struggled to survive, enduring harsh environmental conditions without adequate shelter, food, or clothing. Unsurprisingly, epidemics ravaged these populations during the chaos that followed the war and Reconstruction.[12]

Racism, meanwhile, became reinstitutionalized in new forms. When Reconstruction was defeated in 1877, the Democratic Party, in a compromise with the Republican Party, agreed to elect the Republican candidate Rutherford B. Hayes to the presidency. In return, the Republican Party agreed to give up all attempts to defend the rights of newly freed people in the South.[13] White political hegemony was restored, and, in the words of the famous historian Kenneth Stampp, the South was redeemed. Black codes were introduced, including a system of passes that Black people needed to move about in white areas. Black individuals were forbidden from entering certain professions and from giving testimony against white people, and they were prohibited from owning firearms.

At the same time, a new narrative emerged in white society that the Negro was incapable of surviving outside the confines of slavery. Slavery was recast as a benign institution that provided care and guidance for the Negro. (In case you think that this racist reasoning has been censured and corrected, think again. In 2023, the Florida state education board reintroduced into middle school standards the affirmation that slaves "benefited from slavery by learning valuable skills."[14]) Southern physicians, meanwhile, supported the racial hierarchy of the post–Civil War period with yet more "scientific" and medical explanations to justify keeping Negroes in a state of servitude. Like the slave ship doctors who preceded them, they used health disparities between Black and white populations to "prove" the anatomical and physiological inferiority of the Negro. In 1903, a physician from Pittsburgh named W. T. English argued that the Negro's greater susceptibility to Paget's disease, rickets, hip-joint disease, gigantism, and various psychoses was proof of their physiological inferiority. Another physician, F. Tipton, from Selma, Alabama, claimed that "no amount of charitable aid" could reduce the Negro's "frightful mortality rate."

Southern physicians concluded that Black people could not govern themselves and that they had been better off during slavery. Yet data on slave mortality during the 1850s fails to support the idea that slavery had in any way been beneficial to the enslaved. Things did not get worse for former slaves after slavery was abolished: they stayed exactly the same. The difference in death rates between Black and white populations in the late nineteenth century was the same as that experienced during slavery—and it was still the same in the late twentieth century.[15]

SCIENCE WAS INSTRUMENTALIZED TO PERPETUATE RACISM

Throughout the nineteenth century, arguments about the physiological inferiority of the Negro took new forms as physicians backed up their claims with what they considered to be scientific evidence. Many subscribed to the "Negro extinction hypothesis" developed by the statistician Frederick Hoffman (1865–1946).[16] Hoffman, who went on to become president of the American Statistical Association in 1911, cataloged a variety of sources on morbidity and mortality showing that Negroes experienced higher rates than whites of many infectious diseases (e.g., consumption [tuberculosis], pneumonia, venereal disease, malaria, typhoid, smallpox, measles), behavioral problems (e.g., child neglect, alcoholism, insanity, lunacy), and chronic disease (e.g., cancer). Hoffman argued that these diseases were reducing the reproductive rate of the Negro race such that the Negro would soon become extinct.

Hoffman made no explicitly genetic arguments in his work, but his racist conclusions were in keeping with the popular belief that the condition of Negroes was a result of their innate inferiority. This remained the predominant view of white medicine until the early twentieth century.[17] Twenty years after Hoffman's assertions, Charles B. Davenport, a leading American geneticist, established the Eugenics Record Office (ERO), whose goals included "geneticizing" the inferiority of Negroes and poor whites. The work of the ERO, which operated from 1910 to 1939 in Cold Spring Harbor,

New York, was inspired by the ideas of Sir Francis Galton, a British scientist who believed that inferior genetic stock was out-reproducing superior genetic stock in the human species and that this would result in a condition he called "dysgenesis." Davenport aimed to make the ERO a repository and clearing house for data on human genetic traits that would supply things such as an index of traits in American families and studies of the hereditary consequences of mating. Davenport wanted the ERO to provide advice to Americans on the eugenic fitness of proposed marriages, train fieldworkers to gather data of eugenic importance, encourage the establishment of new centers of eugenics research and education, publish research results, and aid in the dissemination of eugenic "truths." The ERO achieved these goals in spades, including by providing a model eugenic sterilization law that was adopted across the nation, resulting in the forced sterilization of more than sixty-eight thousand Americans by 1968.[18]

Few things illustrate the ERO's work to perpetuate the belief in the innate inferiority of the Negro better than its misrepresentation of the cause of pellagra, a disease rampant in the American South by 1900 whose symptoms include dermatitis, diarrhea, and mental disturbance. Though caused by vitamin deficiency, the ERO conveniently explained it as an inherited genetic disease. When, in 1916, the epidemiologist Joseph Goldberger demonstrated that pellagra was neither caused by an infectious agent nor inherited genetically but rather related to a poor-quality diet, his research was dismissed. Goldberger had noted that no cases of the disease were present among the wealthy and concluded that it was likely related to poverty. To study the disease, he convinced incarcerated volunteers to subsist on a high-carbohydrate diet without protein or fresh green vegetables; within six months, all participants had developed pellagra. Goldberger then demonstrated that he could cure the disease by providing people access to a high-quality balanced diet.[19] His conclusion: if pellagra were properly considered a disease caused by poverty, not genetics, the epidemic could be cured by measures as simple as better jobs and higher wages.

But instead of embracing Goldberger's breakthrough, the ERO lobbied Congress to declare pellagra an inherited genetic disease. As with every other disease associated with poverty, African Americans went on to die at a much higher rate during the pellagra epidemic than European Americans did: through the Great Depression and into the 1940s, the mortality rate of Blacks infected with pellagra was twice that of whites.[20] The ERO's motivation was simple: it wanted Congress's support for its plan to improve the white race through the mandatory eugenic sterilization of various types of so-called defective people.

By the 1960s, while morbidity and mortality rates for biological sources of death were still disproportionately higher in African Americans than in European Americans, African American birth rates had begun surpassing those of European Americans.[21] Because this fact threatened to contradict Hoffman's Negro extinction hypothesis, a new theory was concocted to replace it: the theory of dysgenesis. Arthur Jensen, an educational psychologist at the University of California, Berkeley, claimed that if people with inferior genetic traits (such as Negroes) reproduced at a higher rate than those with superior traits (such as whites), society would eventually collapse under the weight of the genetically unfit.[22]

In the twentieth century, the well-honed practice of attributing the health disparities of African Americans to their physiological inferiority was reinforced with yet more new theories, including the still-accepted belief that African Americans are naturally predisposed to hypertension (high blood pressure). Reports of elevated blood pressure in African Americans began to appear in the 1930s, followed by similar reports about Afro-Caribbean populations in the 1960s. The medical community soon came to believe that hypertension was simply the racial condition of the Negro. In the late 1980s, this conclusion was explained by the "slavery hypertension" hypothesis, according to which Western Africans had evolved the capacity to retain salt in their tissues because salt was rare in Western Africa, an idea reinforced by the deaths that occurred aboard ships during the transatlantic slave trade, specifically during the Middle Passage. In a famous episode of *The Oprah Winfrey Show* from 2007, Oprah Winfrey explains to her guest, Dr. Mehmet Oz, that the enslaved Africans who survived the Middle Passage did so because of a genetic predisposition to retain sodium that was passed on to their offspring. But there is no evidence to support this claim. Salt was abundant in the West African societies that produced enslaved individuals, and there is no way to validate the notion that heat exhaustion was a primary cause of death on slave ships.

The pattern of health disparities between Black and white Americans has continued unbroken into the twenty-first century. In my 2001 book, *The Emperor's New Clothes*, I used data from the National Vital Statistics System to compare patterns of Black and white biological mortality (excluding accidents, homicide, and suicide) by age from three years: 1963, 1980, and 1996. In these years, Black mortality rates among various age groups were 1.3 to 2.5

times greater than white mortality rates. Most strikingly, the largest rates of difference (2.5 times higher) were among the very young (0 to 5 years old) and those in midlife (45 to 55 years old). This means that at those relatively young ages, Blacks were 2.5 times more likely to die from a biological cause than were whites. It's a shocking difference.

The supposed genetic differences of African Americans do nothing to explain these disparities, which are the direct result of the social systems that created and perpetuate them. That means two things: first, these disparities are not random; second, with the right measures, they can be eliminated. Yet physicians continue to believe that Blacks are physiologically destined to live shorter lives than whites. What's worse, this belief blinds physicians and researchers to the real causes of health disparities. These disparities *cannot* be the result of genetic differences between Black and white people for a simple reason: the genetic differences between Black and white people are so minor that they explain *almost nothing* about the differences in how Black Americans get sick or how long they live compared with white Americans.

WHY TWENTY-FIRST-CENTURY DOCTORS ARE STILL GETTING RACE WRONG

I wrote this book to put to rest any assumptions that these dramatic differences in health and longevity are the result of the small amount of genetic difference that exists between African and European Americans. Once I began to study and write about biological and social conceptions of race in the late 1990s, it became apparent to me why, for most of its history, medicine has gotten race wrong. The medical profession, like every other profession in our society, came into being in a context of unquestioned white supremacy. Because of this, it's easy to see where the racist thinking of physicians like Benjamin Rush, Samuel Cartwright, and F. Tipton comes from. What is harder to explain is why racist assumptions persist and continue to hurt the Black population to this day. Because they do.

As an African American, I have experienced racist assumptions directly and watched members of my own family suffer and die because of them. For example, like many former athletes, I have a knee problem caused by repeated injury and exacerbated by age. By 2017, I couldn't climb stairs or walk from my car to my office without cringing in pain. Yet I endured more than three more years of excruciating pain before I was given an artificial knee. During that time, even though I desperately needed surgery, doctors kept repeating the same mantra to me to explain why they kept putting off surgery: they wanted to try everything else they could think of before giving me a knee replacement. It was as if they couldn't see the pain on my face at every appointment.

I might have accepted the doctors' words if—like so many of my friends and relatives—my faith in getting proper medical treatment hadn't already been diminished by experiencing racial discrimination all my life. One example of this is the belief that Blacks feel pain less acutely than whites. The result of that belief is that less pain medication is prescribed to Black than to white patients. And this is only one of many medical misconceptions about Black people that refuses to die. According to a paper published in the *Journal of the American Medical Association*, over the last two decades, racialized medicine has resulted in an excess 1.6 million Black deaths, costing the nation $238 billion in 2018 alone.[23]

The problem is *not* that individual doctors are racist. Some undoubtedly are, but the vast majority of physicians in America today would claim that they are opposed to racism. Most of the doctors that my colleague Andrea Deyrup, a pathologist at Duke University, and I have spoken to over the last few years are horrified to think that racist ideas still exist within a profession whose core principle is "do no harm." What's more, modern medicine prides itself on the principle of being rooted in scientific research.

The problem is that modern medicine has grown out of an age-old system of beliefs rooted squarely in racist assumptions that have worked their way into every corner of the medical world and into the very fabric of American medicine. And this happened because medicine grew more from beliefs than it did from science. In the nineteenth century, it was still common for physicians to bleed people to "balance their humors," and medical leech therapy was widely used to balance humors in Europe and the United States in 1850.[24] The scientific principles that we take for granted today were not widely accepted before the twentieth century (e.g., blood circulation, the germ theory of disease). America didn't have national standards for medical training until well into the twentieth century, and the salaries of medical professors depended on the number of students that they trained. Thus, it's fair to conclude that a great deal of variability existed in the skills and knowledge of physicians.[25]

But to understand how assumptions about the medical "differences" of African Americans became so deeply engrained and why they persist, we must understand how they were built into medicine over time. Views of human variation in the nineteenth century had more to do with theology than science.[26] Even at the beginning of the twentieth century, theories of human variation were based on a belief in creationism: the idea that all humans were the result of a supernatural act of creation and that all their attributes were determined by God. Of course, God in this theory was a white guy, and Jesus was routinely depicted as having European features. The combination of theology and science to try to understand nature was dubbed "natural theology," a widely accepted philosophy according to which all things in nature were a result of God's plan. Many early-twentieth-century white Europeans believed that God had planned for them to dominate the world, and since most physicians in this period were white Christians, the Negro was viewed as physiologically and mentally inferior.

To be fair, until the late nineteenth century, medicine did not have any tools to understand human biological variation that were better than theology. Physicians carried out their work under "typological" concepts of biology according to which all things, including living things, are fixed and unchanging. This notion goes back to the ancient Greeks, including Plato and Aristotle, and was expressed in the Bible in Genesis 1:21: "So God created great creatures of the sea and every living and moving thing with which the water teems, according to their kinds."

Typological thinking in biology was overturned by the arrival of Charles Darwin's theory of evolution by natural selection in the late nineteenth century. But even when it became accepted, evolutionary science faced steep obstacles when it came to changing assumptions about human variation. Western societies in the nineteenth century were so rigidly stratified by socially defined race that Charles Darwin chose *not* to include a discussion of human evolution in the first edition of *On the Origin of Species*, published in 1859. Darwin did not take on the issue of the evolution of human races until 1871, when he published *The Descent of Man, and Selection in Relation to Sex*. In that work, Darwin argued that there was only one human species and that all existing humans shared a recent common ancestry. He also showed that humans were far more alike than they were different.

Unfortunately, most people came to understand evolution not through the writings of Darwin but rather those of one of his contemporaries, Herbert Spencer, a philosopher, psychologist, biologist, sociologist, and anthropologist who distorted Darwin's ideas and coined the expression "survival of the fittest." (Spencer's ideas—along with those of two of the founders of American sociology, Lester Ward [1841–1913] and William Graham Sumner [1840–1910]—were behind the Negro extinction hypothesis.)

CHALLENGES TO THE RACIAL HIERARCHY
BEING IGNORED TO THIS DAY

Individuals who challenged racial hierarchy with scientific knowledge—or mere critical skills—were systematically ignored and dismissed. While the unification of population genetics with natural selection, known as the "neo-Darwinian synthesis," in the early twentieth century offered a fuller understanding of how genetic variation accumulated in populations, anyone who contradicted widely help assumptions about race saw their work challenged and dismissed. In his 1942 book, *Man's Most Dangerous Myth: The Fallacy of Race*, the British anthropologist Ashley Montagu showed why the human species could not be apportioned into biological races.[27] He also explained how natural selection had acted on various human traits in ways such that physical and physiological traits could not be correlated (i.e., one couldn't make conclusions based on the color of a person's skin about other traits such as hair color or intelligence). However, *Man's Most Dangerous Myth* did not revolutionize the medical understanding of anatomy and disease—primarily because it was published while the Nazis and their allies were deploying their racial ideology for medical experimentation and genocide on an unparalleled scale.[28] It is more than ironic that while my father landed on Utah Beach to help put down Nazi racism in 1944, the US Army Medical Corps insisted on maintaining racially segregated blood supplies.[29]

I don't want to sound like I'm excusing the people who crafted racist ideas over the course of history or the medical professionals who embraced those ideas. My goal is to explain how racial fallacies still contribute to racial disparities in health outcomes and why, as a result, Black people die sooner than white people. To overcome these disparities, we must recognize *how* racial misconceptions entered the medical field and understand *why* they persist. Medicine was born and developed in the context of white supremacy and structural racism, and misconceptions about African Americans have literally been built into the medical system over centuries. These ideas are deep rooted, persistent, insidious, and harmful, and we can't eliminate them unless we recognize them for what they are: historically inherited, persistent falsehoods. Students who begin medical school are not required to recognize and respond to the racial smog they inhabit. That means that they will probably never get around to recognizing the fallacies of the racial ideas that they will bring into their own medical practices.

I wrote this book to demonstrate once and for all that the health disparities of African Americans are not the result of genetic differences between socially defined racial groups. Recognizing this is the first step toward creating a society in which everyone can get at least their "three score and ten" and improving the life span and health of all Americans.

To do that, we must understand what evolution is and what it does—and does not—explain about human beings. In the late twentieth century, although doubt was being cast on the idea of classifying the human species into biological races, the medical community continued to ignore how evolutionary biology contributed to the understanding of disease.[30] The only evolutionary concepts that would significantly affect medicine at the time were microbial evolution and antibiotic resistance.[31] As I write this, most physicians still do not understand that all diseases have both evolutionary (ultimate) and physiological, cellular, and molecular (proximate) bases.[32] Part of the explanation for this is that evolutionary biology is not a required course for entry into medical training. And even when it is taught, the need to understand human biological variation from an evolutionary perspective is rarely emphasized.[33]

As you will see in the following chapters, a widespread understanding of evolutionary biology can put an end to the racist assumptions that infect medicine. While the importance of evolutionary biology has been increasingly recognized over the past three decades, few in the field of evolutionary medicine have advanced this perspective as essential to overcoming racial misconceptions in biomedical research and clinical practice as I have.[34]

In part I, I explain why misconceptions in modern medicine born in nineteenth-century typology persist. I discuss how racial injustice causes health injustice (chapter 1) and how a lack of appreciation for the evolutionary causes of disease misdirects both biomedical research and clinical treatment, making it impossible for practitioners to find their way through racial misconceptions (chapter 2).

Part II focuses on the harm that racial medicine has caused and continues to cause, particularly in hypertension and cardiovascular disease (chapter 3), the microbiome (chapter 4), infectious disease (chapter 5), sickle cell anemia (chapter 6), cancer (chapter 7), and the epigenome (chapter 8).

In part III, I describe how to fix the problem, explaining how precision medicine is overpromising its abilities (chapter 10) and discussing how we can change medical minds (chapter 11). In the conclusion, I propose a vision of a world free of racial medicine and racism in medicine, one where we can all live well.

PART I

Why

Chapter One

RACIAL INJUSTICE CAUSES HEALTH INJUSTICE

As it has throughout human history, a person's position in their society powerfully predicts well-being, particularly health and ultimately lifespan. Not everyone gets their threescore and ten, and those who do often spend their later years dying painfully from the cost of surviving their earlier ones. During my undergraduate years, I often received calls from home informing me of the death of an aunt, uncle, or cousin. This was not unexpected given my large extended family. My mother was from a family of eleven and my father from a family of eight. Yet many of those deaths were premature. We understood early death as being expected for those who had survived Jim Crow segregation and for those who had worked in difficult jobs that required consistent exposure to toxic materials. It is surprising that my mother made it in to her eighties given that she worked during the day cleaning rich folks' homes and pulled a second shift at night in a plastics factory. I worked in the same plant as a student, and the experience of choking on plastics fumes during an eight-hour shift was all the incentive I needed to finish college.

It may not be obvious that a person's social status determines how long they will live. However, this has been true since humans formed social hierarchies after the introduction of agriculture and the transition away from the hunter–gatherer lifestyle. This principle is well illustrated by the way that the global pandemic of human immunodeficiency virus (HIV) and acquired immunodeficiency virus (AIDS) unfolded in the latter portion of the twentieth century. When people first began to contract HIV and AIDS, it was as if the disease had appeared out of nowhere. In the United States, HIV and AIDS rapidly became epidemic in the gay male community. Some evangelical preachers, such as Billy Graham, claimed that the disease was a curse from God to punish the sin of homosexuality.[1]

The virus was not a curse, nor was its origin particularly mysterious. Like many pathogenic viruses, the human immunodeficiency virus (HIV) originated in another species, in this case, chimpanzees or possibly gorillas (HIV-1) and monkeys (HIV-2).[2] This origin is inferred from the similarity of HIV genome sequences to simian immunodeficiency virus (SIV). An important difference, however, is that over time, SIV evolved lower virulence (i.e., a reduced ability to make the host sick) in apes and monkeys, thus causing little disease in those species. This is because the SIV virus had been present in these species for much longer, for thousands of years at least. On the other hand, the best estimates of when HIV-1 crossed over into humans is on the order of eighty years ago.[3] This transmission occurred somewhere in Central Africa, with the earliest known samples of HIV-1 coming from patients from Kinshasa, Democratic Republic of the Congo, in 1959 and 1960.[4]

It is common for viruses to shift host species, and the more closely related host species are, the more likely it is that the virus will jump between those species. This is because viruses use a type of protein expressed on the surface of host cells to facilitate entry into them. Proteins from closely related species share more of their component amino acids in common, thus also sharing more of their three-dimensional shapes. For example, the amino acid sequence of the angiotensin-converting enzyme 2 (ACE2) receptor in mammals is highly conserved. Therefore, it didn't take a whole lot of evolution for severe acute respiratory syndrome (SARS) viruses from nonhuman mammals to be able to use the human receptor.

The recent COVID-19 pandemic most likely arose from a strain of the SARS coronavirus (SARS-CoV) that had been replicating in bats or pangolins or from a recombinant of viruses from both species.[5] The shift to a new host often comes with an increase in virulence since the new host has not yet evolved resistance to the virus. Subsequent virus evolution in the new host can thus result in either the evolution of greater virulence or greater transmission. Virulence and transmission often trade off against each other, as when the original SARS-CoV-2 variants that emerged had strong virulence but were later outpaced by the Omicron strain, which had lower virulence but greater transmissibility.[6]

However, in the case of HIV transmission in humans, there has been no shift in virulence for transmissibility. This has in part resulted from differences in the way the viruses are transmitted. SARS-CoV-2 is airborne, whereas HIV is transmitted mainly through sexual contact. HIV's primary adaptation in humans seems to have been the evolution of dormancy after an initial bout of severe symptoms. This adaptation allows the virus to spread via sex between an infected person (who may not know that they have HIV) and an uninfected partner. Even though HIV can be spread through infected blood supplies, transmission occurs primarily via sexual activity. In most of the world, HIV transmission occurs via men having sex with men. In 2012, in North and South America, Western and Eastern Europe, the Middle East, Asia, and Australia, it was found that more men were being infected with HIV than women.[7] However, Africa showed the opposite pattern—with more women being infected than men—indicating that most HIV transmission in African countries resulted from infected men having sex with uninfected women.

To understand how this gendered pattern emerged, we must first understand how the apartheid labor system operated. This system, implemented by the Boer and English rulers of South Africa in 1948, seized the nation's most valuable land and resources for the white minority, relegating the Indigenous Africans to barren tribal homelands. Africans could seek labor in white South Africa, where women were employed mainly as domestics and men mostly in industry and mining. Men were isolated from their wives or domestic partners for months. Around the mines, brothels sprang up, providing workers with access to sex, drugs, and alcohol.[8] This resulted in a few sex workers infecting hundreds, if not thousands, of patrons. In the 1940s, a rural doctor named Sidney Kark demonstrated that the workers' circular migration pattern (from homeland to mine to homeland) was responsible for a syphilis epidemic associated with the diamond mines and tribal homelands. The harsh conditions of the mines, causing many workers to experience malnutrition and exhaustion, predisposed miners to infection. The same conditions led to the spread of HIV infection throughout South Africa, which in turn led to the spread of the disease across the region and then the continent.[9] The spread of HIV was also facilitated by the relative powerlessness of women in the societies that furnished the migrant workers of South Africa. Wives and girlfriends were often forced to have sex with men whom they knew were infected.[10]

The apartheid labor system and Africa's widespread poverty led to a rapid spread of the disease across the continent, such that in 2012, more than

23 million sub-Saharan Africans were living with HIV or AIDS. This is in stark comparison to the much lower numbers in Southeast Asia (4 million), North America (1.4 million), South America (1.4 million), Eastern Europe (1.4 million), and Western Europe (0.9 million). The smaller number of cases in these countries can also be attributed to the fact that transmission there was driven more by men having sex with men rather than the primarily heterosexual transmission in Africa. Thus, in 2012, 84 percent of adult deaths due to HIV and AIDS, 91 percent of HIV and AIDS infections in children, and 94 percent of child deaths due to HIV and AIDS occurred in sub-Saharan Africa. Further, 95 percent of the children orphaned by HIV and AIDS lived in in sub-Saharan Africa. In 2010, an estimated 40 million African children had been orphaned by HIV and AIDS.[11] These numbers illustrate the dramatic impact of HIV and AIDS on Africa as compared with other regions of the world. This pandemic did not occur because Africans are somehow more genetically vulnerable to the disease. Rather, it occurred because of the historical legacies of colonialism, modern-day imperialism, and the resultant and ongoing underdevelopment of African countries.

DISEASE CLASSIFICATION

To understand how structural racism makes people sick, we must first understand the categories of disease that can exist in a species. Modern medicine tends to classify disease by the anatomical or physiological system affected as opposed to the evolutionary, genetic, and physiological reasons that a disease exists. For example, *Robbins & Kumar Basic Pathology* (now in its eleventh edition, for which I was a consultant) is one of the most widely used texts in medical schools around the world.[12] Its chapters cover diseases of the immune system, blood vessels, heart, lung, kidney, liver and gallbladder, pancreas, and skin. The approach used to understand these diseases focuses on cellular and molecular mechanisms. Evolutionary biologists would characterize this approach as focusing on proximate mechanisms. Essentially, this way of thinking asks what in an organism's system causes the malfunction that results in disease.

While such investigations are important, they do not tell us everything we need to know. Specifically, why does a particular disease exist, and why are some populations more likely to suffer from a particular disease? To answer these questions, we must take an evolutionary (or ultimate) approach. Such an approach considers all features of an organism (both good and bad) to be the result of evolution via natural selection. Thus, an understanding of how evolution operated to allow a given disease to exist can provide powerful insights to improve treatment for that disease. In the evolutionary classification of disease, genetic and physiological causes take precedence. This classification consists of seven causal categories, of which diseases can be influenced by more than one.

1. Diseases with Genetic Causes

When most people think about genetic diseases, they invariably racialize them. This is true of physicians as well.[13] "Sickle cell anemia is a Black disease." "Only white people get cystic fibrosis." "American Indians get diabetes." And so on. Genetic diseases get racialized because most people still believe that humans have biological races and that these races differ genetically in ways that determine their health and disease profiles.[14] However, the races we understand in American life are socially defined and not accurate descriptors of human biological variation. Any two people on the planet chosen at random will share anywhere from 99.4 to 99.9 percent of their genome in common. This means that most genetic variants are found all over the globe but in different frequencies by population. (In chapter 4, I take a deep dive into how this variation in frequency plays a role in determining the prevalence of sickle cell anemia.)

Genes determine phenotypes (physical traits) differentially depending on whether the trait in question (in this case, disease) is caused by a single or several genes of high penetrance or influenced by many genes. Single-gene disease traits in humans are cataloged in the Online Mendelian Inheritance in Man (OMIM) database.[15] Its entries are comprehensive and include the location of the variant in the human genome, as well as the name of the locus. Information is also provided in categories including description, clinical features, biochemical features, inheritance, cytogenetics, population genetics, molecular genetics, genotype/phenotype correlations, pathogenesis, animal models, history, and references. I have never found a genetic disease in this database limited to one socially defined race. For example, the OMIM population genetics entry for Hutchinson-Gilford progeria syndrome, a disease that mimics premature aging, reports the prevalence of the disease as one per eight million newborns in the United States and one per four million in the Netherlands. It also states that cases have been reported on all continents and in all ethnicities. The prevalence of this disease is so low because those who carry the genetic trait rarely live past the age of thirteen and almost never reproduce. This means that the gene can appear in a population only by a mutation event, and the frequency of such events in populations is random. Mutation rates are pretty standard across human populations, ranging between 10^{-8} and 10^{-7} substitutions per base pair per generation.[16] Thus, all genetic diseases that significantly impair survival and reproduction are rare worldwide.

The frequency of phenylketonuria (PKU), a serious genetic disorder that prevents the breakdown of the amino acid phenylalanine (MIM ID no. 261600), is 8.4×10^{-6} in Japanese people, 6.25×10^{-5} in Chinese people, and 2.0×10^{-4} in Irish, Scottish, and Yemenite Jewish people.[17] To get a sense of what these frequencies look like, imagine that you have a collection of a million marbles, some white, representing the functional gene, and some red, representing the nonfunctional gene that causes phenylketonuria. In the case of the Japanese sample, there would be about eight red marbles and 999,992 white marbles, whereas in the Chinese sample, you would have about six red marbles and 999,994 white marbles. Another study of PKU frequency by socially defined race in Southeast England found a frequency of 1.14×10^{-4} for white people, 1.1×10^{-5} for Black people, and 2.9×10^{-5} for Asian people.[18]

There is no rhyme or reason to the global pattern of this variant, as would be predicted by the interaction of natural selection with the disease and by individual population history via random genetic drift, the random fluctuation of gene frequency owing to small population size. In some cases, modern medical treatments can increase the survival and reproduction of those with a given disease and thus increase its frequency. However, genetic counseling can decrease the frequency of disease-causing genetic variants and thus decrease their frequency in groups in which it was formerly at higher prevalence. In such cases, access to medical care and genetic counseling is the most important determinate in changing prevalence—not genetic ancestry or socially defined race.

There is only one way that natural selection can increase the frequency of a disease-causing allele (an alternative form of a gene): the allele must be beneficial when it is heterozygous, that is, when paired with a different allele a third phenotype is produced. This new phenotype has superior reproductive success compared to either homozygous genotype. People have two alleles for each gene, one received from their mother and one from their father. To display a particular trait, sometimes just one allele is needed (dominant); for some, two of the same allele are needed (recessive).

For example, the gene that causes blue eye color is found on chromosome 15 (*OCA2* found at position 15q13.1), but a person will have blue eyes only if they received the blue eye variant from both parents; that is, they must receive two of the same allele; that is, the alleles are homozygous. In humans, brown eye color is dominant to blue, so a person who received a brown variant from one parent and a blue variant from the other will have brown eyes; that is, the alleles are heterozygous. But alleles often do not show simple dominance; in such cases, a person who received alternative alleles from their parents will display a trait that is intermediate between the two. This occurs in sickle cell anemia. A person without the sickle cell variant will have normally shaped red blood cells that carry oxygen effectively, and a person who received the sickle cell variant from both parents will have red blood cells that are severely sickled and deficient in their capacity to carry oxygen. However, a person with one "normal" allele and one sickle cell allele will have partially sickled red blood cells. The capacity of the person's red blood cells to carry oxygen will be less than that of a person without the sickle cell trait, but this is balanced by the fact that malaria parasites cannot invade those cells. So, people who are heterozygous for the sickle cell variant typically show greater survivorship (i.e., they live longer) than those who are not in areas with high rates of malarial transmission.

This is called heterozygote advantage, and it explains the high frequency we observe of alleles that are deleterious when homozygous (e.g., variants that produce sickle cell hemoglobin, as will be discussed in chapter 4). Another case of heterozygote advantage occurs in ovalocytosis, a disease whose high prevalence is Southeast Asia is also driven by heterozygote advantage against malaria.[19] Homozygous individuals have a severe blood cell disorder, which in usually fatal in utero without extreme medical intervention, but, as with sickle cell anemia, heterozygous individuals show superior survivorship against malaria.

Whereas natural selection generally does not increase the frequency of disease-causing alleles, genetic drift often does. As mentioned earlier, genetic drift is the random change in allele frequency that occurs when a population is dramatically reduced in size. This occurs in humans as a result of both natural disasters and intentional actions to destroy particular racial or cultural groups, that is, genocide. In an example of the consequences of a natural event, at least one of the male survivors of a typhoon in the Pingelapese archipelago in 1780 carried a loss-of-function mutation in the *CNGA3* gene. This mutation results in a type of color blindness caused by a dysfunction in the cone photoreceptors of the eye and is displayed in 4 to 10 percent of the archipelago's current residents. However, the worldwide occurrence of this kind of color blindness is just one in thirty thousand individuals—about 0.003 percent.[20] Natural disasters that dramatically reduce human population sizes (with survivorship having nothing to do with genetics) have occurred throughout the history our species.

Conversely, genocide is a relatively new behavior of our species, dating back only to the nineteenth century. While there is considerable debate over the meaning of the term, for my purposes, the 1948 United Nations Genocide Convention definition will suffice: "acts with intent to destroy, in whole or in part, a national, ethnic, racial, or religious group."[21] There is little doubt that the actions of the United States government against the Indigenous peoples of North America over the last 250 years or so meet this definition. Several cases support this claim, including that of the Navajo people interned at Fort Defiance in Arizona from 1863 to 1868 who were forced to leave their traditional lands, making arduous treks of hundreds of miles, including the "Long Walk" to Fort Sumner in New Mexico Territory.[22] About ten thousand Navajo people began the journey to the New Mexico camp, but only about eight thousand are thought to have survived.[23] From that small population, the Navajo now number about 330,000. Similarly, owing to actions of the US government, the Jicarilla Apache declined to a population of only about six hundred in the early twentieth century and now number just 3,300.[24]

Both the Navajo and Jicarilla Apache peoples, who are Athabascan-language speakers, have a very high prevalence of a disorder known as severe combined immunodeficiency, Athabascan type (SCIDA). The variety found in these groups results in a lack of T, B, and NK cells, which are key components of the immune response. The prevalence of this condition in the general population is 1/1,000,000 but 1/2,000 in the Navajo and Apache peoples. SCIDA results from a nonsense mutation in the *DCLRE1C* gene, which abrogates the function of a protein (Artemis) involved in DNA repair and the recombination required to make a necessary protein involved in the immune response.[25] The 1/1,000,000 frequency of affected individuals worldwide indicates that the frequency of this variant in humans is determined by a balance between mutation and selection. Because people with the condition rarely reproduce, the only way that the variant can appear in a population is through a new mutation. In the case of the survivors of the genocidal actions taken against the Navajo and Apache nations, by simple chance, carriers of the SCIDA variant were elevated by orders of magnitude resulting in the disproportionate prevalence of this disease in these groups.

Diseases with Complex Genetic Origins

The remaining six causal categories of the evolutionary classification of disease involve diseases with complex genetic origins. Diseases such as cancer, diabetes, heart disease, and stroke result from the actions of many genes from across the genome. Such traits will show a continuous distribution of phenotypes (as opposed to the limited phenotypic ratios produced by traits produced by one gene [1:2:1] or two genes [9:3:3:1]). The shape of quantitative distributions for such traits is often that of the normal (or bell) curve. For example, a trait determined by five genetic loci in which both parents are heterozygous would display eleven phenotypic classes in the offspring, with the ratio of individuals shown in figure 1.1. The more genes that contribute to a trait, the more the distribution of the trait will approach a continuous normal distribution. For example, the human life span is determined by virtually all protein-coding genes in the human genome, of which there are about nineteen thousand. Figure 1.2 shows data for the distribution of human life spans in the United States from the year 2020. This data is skewed to the left because humans are living longer than ever before; however, it still shows the continuous distribution expected of a trait determined by many genes.

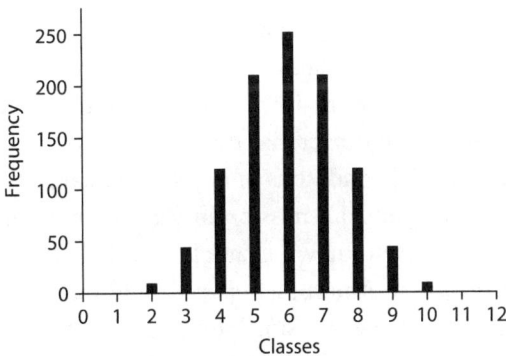

FIGURE 1.1. Frequency distribution for the phenotype produced by the action of 5 genetic loci. There are 11 classes, and a total of 1,024 individuals. The ratio expected of the most extreme phenotypes is 1/1024 (class 1 and class 11).

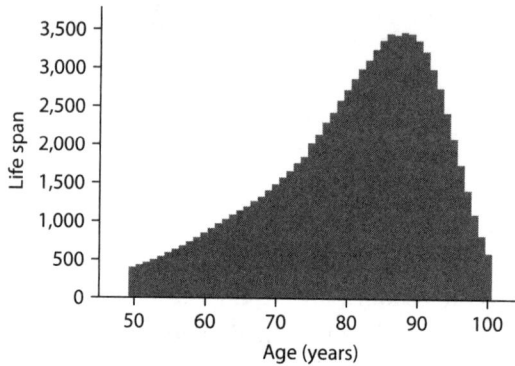

FIGURE 1.2. Frequency distribution for life span in the United States in 2020.

2. DISEASES WITH ENVIRONMENTAL CAUSES

Organisms are in a constant struggle to maintain their physiological function against various components of their physical and social environments.
These struggles include gathering enough nourishment and water, preventing heat and cold stress, maintaining oxygen levels, and avoiding predation
and infection. Throughout much of the existence of our species, infectious
disease has been a significant cause of morbidity and mortality. Environmental causes of illness include a wide variety of pathogens that infect humans:
viruses, bacteria, and unicellular and multicellular eukaryotes (organisms
with complex cellular structures). Human activity has played a crucial role
in creating environments that make pathogens so successful. For example, it
is thought that malaria evolved the capacity to infect humans as a result of
both the domestication of animals and the crowding of humans into settle-
ments, making transmission easier.[26] These conditions worked the same
way in facilitating viral and bacterial transmission. What is not generally
understood is how social conditions of oppression played a role in the differential rates of pathogen transmission in various communities throughout human history. A well-known example of this is the transmission of
smallpox by Europeans to Amerindian populations in the seventeenth century, such as that causing the 1616 smallpox epidemic in New England. Such
epidemics had both a genetic (lower HLA genetic diversity in Amerindian
populations via the founder effect) and a social component (disruption of
Amerindian societies because of warfare against them). In another example,

during the time of American chattel slavery, even though enslaved West Africans had various antimalarial adaptations, they still died from malaria at differentially higher rates because of exposure, poor nutrition, and over-work resulting from their enslaved condition.[27] The early differential in COVID-19 infections among African Americans and Latin Americans in the United States was driven by environmental conditions such as crowding and being unable to work from home.[28]

Environments also play a key role in complex disease. In 2019, the leading complex biological causes of death in the United States were heart disease, cancers, respiratory disease, and cerebrovascular disease.[29] In economically privileged nations, heart disease is an archetypical case of environmental mismatch. Well-known environmental and behavioral risk factors include poor diet, sedentarism, ambient air and noise pollution, sleep deprivation, and psychosocial stress (which is primarily environmental), as well as body composition, cardiovascular fitness, muscle strength, and the functionality of the intestinal microbiome (which may be influenced as much by genetic as by environmental factors). Strong evidence suggests that psychosocial stress resulting from structural racism differentially predisposes African Americans to heart disease (as will be discussed in chapter 8).[30] One recent study found higher levels of CpG methylation in promoter regions of metabolic genes associated with heart muscle failure among Black men with low socio-economic status, a population that has been negatively affected by socially defined race.[31] Methylation influences patterns of gene expression, thus in this case environmental influences on methylation results in dysregulation of metabolism causing disease. Thus, the historical presence of structural racism in America (both a social and physical environmental factor) is consistent with the long-standing disparity in heart disease by socially defined race.

3. DISEASES OF HOMEOSTASIS

Homeostasis is the ability of an organism to maintain a stable internal physiological environment even as external conditions change. Diseases of homeostasis affect physiological systems that evolved to be plastic and adjustable. For example, if our blood pressure rises too high, we are in danger of an embolism (stroke); if it drops too low, we may go into cardiac arrest. The dysregulation of our steady states can have both genetic and environmental causes. These causes are particularly revealed by the evolutionary mismatch in which all modern humans exist. *Evolutionary mismatch* refers to the fact that our basic physiology evolved more than three hundred thousand years ago when our ancestors were hunter-gatherers in Africa. The rate of genetic change within our species was much slower than the rate of cultural change in our societies. This means that our basic physiological systems are greatly challenged in the novel environments that exist in modern industrial societies. These new environments often cause an inappropriate adjustment of our homeostatic set points.

Phenotypic (physical) plasticity is the developmental counterpart of adjustable homeostatic set points.[32] For example, it has been recently demonstrated that cellular plasticity can be observed in almost all cell types within the adult pancreas.[33] In this case, cellular plasticity occurs when the pancreas is presented with various types of stress stimuli. It occurs in various cell types within the pancreas and by various molecular mechanisms. The plasticity allows both pancreatic and nonpancreatic cells to be harnessed in the generation of new insulin-producing beta cells. Insulin is the hormone that regulates glucose concentration in the bloodstream and is involved in glucose storage in the liver, muscle, and adipose tissue. Phenotypic plasticity affecting the pancreas of growing children undoubtedly results from diets dominated by ultra-processed foods, which in turn have been linked to increasing rates of childhood obesity, particularly among the poor of Western societies.[34] Importantly, poverty and socially defined race in the United States are intimately related.

Both adjustable homeostasis and phenotypic plasticity allow for the flexibility required to deal with variable environments. However, both mechanisms allow for physiological systems to be fixed in the wrong state. Diseases of homeostasis include substance use disorders, obesity, type 2 diabetes, atherosclerosis, hypertension, and cardiovascular disease. All are influenced by social determinants, again resulting in differential prevalences by socially defined race.

4. DISEASES RESULTING FROM LACK OF MAINTENANCE

The evolutionary basis of aging is conserved in all animals and results from the declining force of natural selection on the age of the adult somatic tissue.[35] Somatic tissue is responsible for the physiological functions that keep an organism alive (such as muscles, nervous, skin). This is contrasted to germ tissue which is responsible for the production of reproductive cells (ovaries, testes). This can be explained in the context of the human life

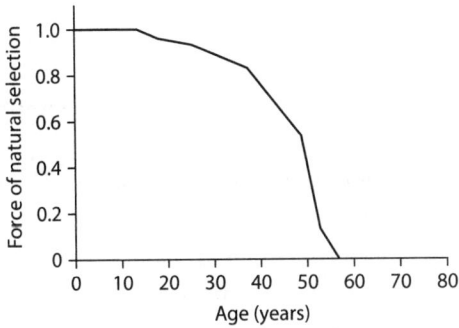

FIGURE 1.3. The declining force of natural selection with age

course. Natural selection acts most powerfully to remove any genetic variant that negatively affects the fertilization and development of an embryo (from conception to birth). It is also at maximum power to remove any genetic variant that negatively affects growth from birth to the age of first reproduction (for humans, this is about thirteen years of age). The force against genetic variants that negatively affect the reproductive period of life declines across the reproductive period, dropping to zero at the point at which the possibility of reproduction has ceased (figure 1.3). In brief, this means that natural selection is unable to remove genes whose negative effects occur after the possibility of reproduction has ceased in a species. This also means that we evolved to perpetuate our genomes across generations, not necessarily to extend our lifespans. Our developmental and reproductive systems illustrate this: we are at our best physiologically during our growth and reproductive years.

The population genetic mechanisms that govern the evolution of aging are mutation accumulation and antagonistic pleiotropy (refers to a gene that is beneficial in early life but detrimental to survival in late life, discussed further in chapter 2). *Mutation accumulation* refers to the fact that genes with no negative impact on our survival or reproduction during our development and reproductive periods will accumulate in populations by genetic drift. Mutation accumulation and antagonistic pleiotropy have also been demonstrated to account for aging in a variety of experimental organisms. For example, whole-genome sequencing of fruit flies exhibiting postponed senescence (aging) shows starkly different patterns of single-nucleotide variation between early-reproduced (high early fecundity, short life) and delayed-reproduced (low early fecundity, long life) *Drosophila melanogaster*.[36] My own work showed that these mechanisms persisted in replicated experiments and provided additional genetic mechanisms (indels, transposable genetic elements) that were operating to control the pattern of aging.[37]

An example of mutation accumulation in humans is Huntington's disease (also known as Huntington's chorea). Huntington's disease is a neurodegenerative disease caused by a dominant mutation in the HTT locus that encodes the huntingtin protein. This mutation is a series of nucleotide insertions (CAG_n). The CAG triplet encodes the amino acid glutamine, and the more insertions there are, the more dysfunctional the protein becomes and the worse the disease becomes. The length of the insertions determines the age of onset of the condition. Huntington's typically manifests after reproductive age; however, longer repeats cause the disease to emerge in adolescence (this occurs in less than 10 percent of Huntington's cases). Very long insertions result in death in utero; thus, across generations, the disease can disappear from families if those carrying the trait are never born.

As the short repeat genes have no impact on survival or reproductive success, their frequency in populations worldwide is very low; in Western countries, the prevalence is 3–7/100,000 individuals. However, since the frequency of this disease operates by genetic drift, prevalence is highly variable. For example, the prevalence in African Americans in South Carolina is only 0.5/100,000 people, compared to about 15/100,000 for African Americans as a whole; other estimates are 3.8/100,000 in Japan, 0.6/100,000 in South Africa, and 0.5/100,000 in Finland.[38]

However, it is important to understand that not all variants governed by mutation accumulation are associated with severe disease at later ages. Most operate by subtle but cumulative effects on the dysregulation of cellular or molecular function as we age. The proximate mechanisms associated with aging are multiform, occurring at the physiological, cellular, and molecular levels (e.g., wear and tear, hormonal controls, oxidative stress, somatic mutation, DNA methylation).[39] Diseases that result from lack of maintenance include neurodegeneration, cancers, osteoporosis, cardiovascular disease, type 2 diabetes, and arthritis. As with diseases of homeostasis, the prevalence of these conditions is influenced by both genetic and environmental factors. Recent studies have shown that mutation accumulation also influences aging in humans (as will be discussed in chapter 2).

The diversity of age-related diseases associated with mutation accumulation is unsurprising simply because of the sheer numbers of genetic variants that display neutrality in early life. The impact of these variants differs by population, however, as their frequency is also determined by genetic drift. Thus, a study of mutation accumulation variants associated with disease in later life generated from a European population might not be replicated entirely for populations from Africa or Asia—or for the Finnish population, whose allele frequencies were largely determined by genetic drift.

Variants governed by antagonistic pleiotropy should be found at high frequency in all human populations. This is because such variants are favored by natural selection because they improve the likelihood of survival in early life and reproduction at the cost of survival in later life. In short, natural selection increases the frequency of "good" genes and eliminates "bad" ones. Thus, antagonistic pleiotropy is the most insidious of the population genetic mechanisms accounting for aging because it results from natural selection favoring "good" genes. This is because the beneficial character of these variants in early life means that positive natural selection will drive them to fixation in the population (meaning that every person in the population will have them). Evidence for the role of the antagonistic pleiotropy mechanism in human aging will be discussed in chapter 2.

For the reasons cited here, it is highly unlikely that the differences in prevalence that we see in age-related conditions governed by antagonistic pleiotropy across populations have a genetic basis. In other words, the differential patterns of age-associated disease across socially defined racial groups are not driven primarily by genetic differences.

5. DISEASES THAT ARE THE BY-PRODUCTS OF DEFENSE SYSTEMS

These diseases result from how we defend ourselves against pathogens or other environmental insults to our bodies. Defenses always come at a cost; they can be deficient (not work well) or excessive (work too well), or they can simply malfunction. Because defenses also arise from our homeostatic systems, they are also subject to evolutionary mismatch (e.g., dysfunction resulting from a novel environment). The prevalence of these types of diseases in industrialized societies has increased as that of environmentally caused diseases has declined. Examples include autoimmune diseases, allergic diseases, asthma, fibrosis and metaplasia, hemodynamic and thromboembolic diseases, obsessive-compulsive disorder, phobias, paranoias, anxiety, and panic disorders.[40]

As a case in point, the prevalence of allergies and asthma has increased across the industrialized world in conjunction with changes in hygiene.

Asthma is a chronic inflammatory disorder of the airways. It causes recurrent episodes of bronchial spasms that lead to wheezing, breathlessness, chest tightness, and cough (particularly in the early morning and at night). Asthma is characterized by intermittent, reversible airway obstruction, chronic bronchial inflammation, bronchial smooth muscle breakdown and hyperreactivity, and increased mucus secretion.[41] Studies of pediatric asthma examining risk factors associated with socially defined race have found that material hardships (e.g., poor housing quality, housing crowding, lack of amenities, lack of a vehicle) contribute to diagnoses and emergency department visits.[42]

African Americans have experienced poor housing conditions since the time of chattel slavery. W. E. B. Du Bois discussed the poor quality of African Americans' housing in his landmark study of 1899.[43] He showed that Black people paid higher rents for substandard housing and demonstrated a connection between poor housing and social problems (e.g., crime, poverty, disease). The connection between housing quality and neighborhood physical condition continues to this day. These two factors are indicators of a family's purchasing power. For example, when differences in family composition and socioeconomic resources were controlled for, it was found that Black and Hispanic families remained less likely than white families to live in high-quality units and neighborhoods in the 1990s.[44] To this day across the United States, racial minority families are less likely to own their homes.[45]

The low rate of home ownership in racialized communities in the United States has its roots in the late 1930s. That was when the Home Owners' Loan Association began "redlining," that is, refusing to provide money for home loans to those living in areas considered an economic risk. Loans made to individuals who lived in neighborhoods with a high proportion of Whites were considered "secure," whereas loans made to people living in neighborhoods with a high proportion of Blacks or Hispanics were considered "insecure." Such neighborhoods were marked on maps in red (hence "redlining"). Thus, home ownership in redlined neighborhoods was much lower than in others (figure 1.4). The health consequences of redlining persist today. A recent study of eight urban communities in California showed that the relative risk of emergency department visits in formerly redlined communities for asthma was 1.39 compared to nonredlined communities. These communities had higher percentages of Black and Hispanic

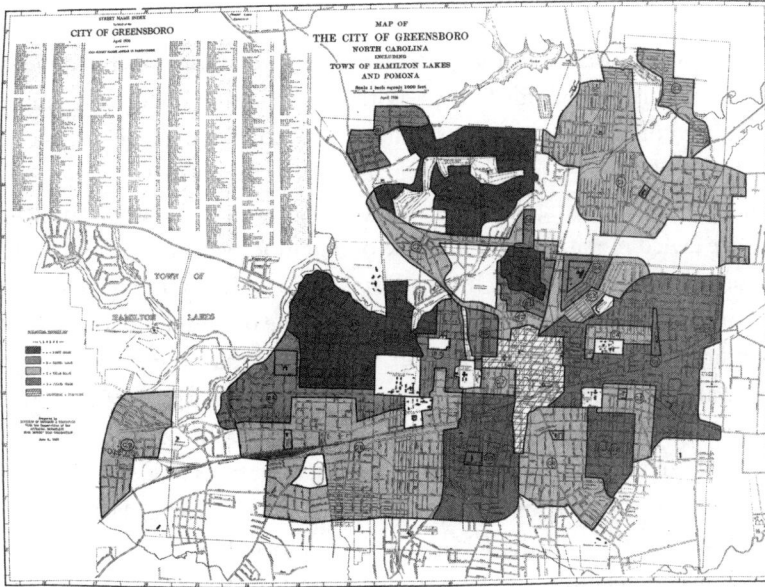

FIGURE 1.4. Redlining: the 1936 Home Owners' Loan Corporation assessment of loan risk in Greensboro, North Carolina. Because of racial segregation in housing, certain areas of Greensboro (the three darker shaded regions at lower right on this map) were occupied disproportionately by African Americans—and still are today. *Source*: Mapping Inequality: Redlining in New Deal America, https://dsl.richmond.edu/panorama/redlining/data/NC-Greensboro#cityData, accessed December 20, 2024.

residents and higher rates of poverty compared with other communities, and they had also been exposed to higher levels of particulate matter from diesel pollution.[46]

Genome-wide analyses of asthma risk variants have identified different loci in African and European Americans (11q21 in African Americans and 6p21 in European Americans).[47] And a more recent study found that percentage of African ancestry is a predictor of the prevalence of nocturnal asthma.[48] However, this study did not examine factors other than ancestry, such as socioeconomic status, exposure to toxic airborne pollutants, cockroach infestation, or material hardship, all of which have been associated with predisposition to asthma. So, once again we are faced with studies that do not examine the lack of environmental equity between the groups being compared and jump to the conclusion that genes are the primary cause of the differences in the prevalence of this disease by socially defined race.

6. DISEASES FROM STOCHASTIC DEVELOPMENTAL PROBLEMS

The word *stochastic* is a just fancy way of saying "chance." Most people have some familiarity with cards or dice. With a fair die, the chance of rolling any particular number is one out of six, or, in probability language, $1/6 = 0.166$. The chance of rolling the same number in a row is $(1/6) \times (1/6) = (1/36) = 0.027$. Errors that occur during the replication of DNA occur by chance. These mistakes are called mutations, and the rate of mutations varies depending on the type of mutation. Generally, in organisms like us, the mutation rate ranges from one per one million (1×10^{-6}) to one per one hundred million (1×10^{-8}) base pairs per genome per generation. A mutation that changes one nucleotide for another is called a single-nucleotide polymorphism (SNP). Even one change in nucleotide sequence can cause a severe problem if it changes the amino acid in the protein sequence. However, mutations that delete or insert nucleotides into a protein-coding sequence are even worse. Mistakes such as inversions, in which the DNA sequence is inserted backward, can also occur. Finally, deletions or duplications of entire chromosomes can occur during gamete formation. These mutations, known as macromutations, have the worst effects. For example, Turner syndrome is a disease affecting only females that results when one of the X chromosomes is missing or partially missing, meaning that a person has forty-five chromosomes instead of forty-six. People with Turner syndrome experience stunted growth and reduced heart and mental function. Their ovaries fail to develop, and their lifespans are about thirteen years shorter than the general population. The prevalence of this condition in the United States over the last few decades has been 3.2/10,000 live births but has been lower in African American and Hispanic women than in European American women.[49] In Canada in 2016, the prevalence of Turner syndrome was 1/2,500 live female births.[50]

The fact that conditions like Turner syndrome result from chance means that there is no consistent pattern of the condition by socially defined race. The most severe of these developmental disorders will occur in populations at the mutation rate. Genetic drift alters the frequency of stochastic developmental phenotypes. For example, the frequency of intersex karyotypes (e.g., Turner syndrome [XO] and Klinefelter syndrome, which occurs when a person assigned male at birth has an extra X chromosome [XXY]) in Indigenous African populations in South Africa is higher than in other African populations.[51]

7. DISEASES RESULTING FROM MATERNAL-PATERNAL
AND MATERNAL-OFFSPRING FITNESS CONFLICTS

Females and males can improve their reproductive success by different means. Generally, the sex that gestates the offspring tends to be more selective in choosing a mate. For example, in sea horses, males gestate the fertilized egg inside their bodies. They are more selective in choosing a female to donate the egg to than females are in choosing a male partner. In species in which females gestate the offspring, females are choosier. Evolution favors the reduction of conflict between males and females in sexual species resulting in an equilibrium in which both partners benefit from the reproductive effort. Also in species in which females gestate the offspring, conflicts arise between the interests of the offspring and those of the mother. For example, a weaning pup that monopolizes its mother's milk supply will grow faster than its siblings, but the mother will want all of its offspring to grow and survive.

The equilibrium of maternal–paternal and maternal–offspring conflicts occur at the species level. For example, invasive placentas are a primitive trait of placental mammals. The hominids have particularly invasive placentation compared to nonhuman primates.[52] Human fetuses can increase their provisioning via expanding spiral arteries and increasing maternal blood pressure. A disruption in this equilibrium can result in dangerously high blood pressure in the mother, as in the condition preeclampsia. Preeclampsia is characterized by a rise in blood pressure during pregnancy that is associated with signs of damage to other organs; it is also a leading cause of premature birth. In this condition, placental blood vessels typically become abnormally narrow, resulting in the increase in blood pressure. The prevalence of preeclampsia in the United States was 2 to 5 percent of live births in 2008. However, there was a notable disparity between African and European American women (49.2/1,000 versus 44.0/1,000).

Given the complexity of the physiological mechanisms involved in preeclampsia, it is clear that genetic, environmental, and chance effects all play a role. A recent meta-analysis examined 9,515 people with the condition and 157,719 without, all of Eurasian descent, for genomic variants associated with risk of preeclampsia.[53] The authors found that only five statistically differentiated SNPs (logp10 > 8) of the 11,796,347 examined accounted for about 0.67 percent of the variance in preeclampsia risk. This means that along the entire human genome, they could only detect five places that in combination explained less than 1% of the risk of developing this disease. The authors suggested that these genetic effects affect both maternal hypertension and body mass index. Thus, this study's findings shows that there is not a strong genetic cause for the disparity in preeclampsia between African and European American women. However, studies of psychosocial stress differences between these two populations and their association with differential rates of preeclampsia are far more promising.[54] Psychosocial stress activates the hypothalamic–pituitary–adrenal axis. This is the brain system that responds to perceived stress and modulates our physiology by inducing the secretion of corticotrophin, which in turn is associated with systemic inflammation known to be a risk factor for preeclampsia. Numerous studies have shown that African American women experience higher levels of psychosocial stress than do European Americans.[55] However, at least one study has shown that controlling for psychosocial risk reduces but does not completely eliminate the difference in preeclampsia incidence between these groups.[56] Thus, preeclampsia results from a defense system (inflammation) causing disruption of the maternal–fetal fitness equilibrium.

RACISM AS THE ROOT CAUSE OF HEALTH DISPARITY

The classification of disease in the context of evolutionary (or ultimate) and proximate (i.e., genetic, physiological, cellular, and molecular) causes provides a powerful tool to elucidate how racism operates to create health disparities. I came to this recognition early on in my career.[57] Individual diseases often result from a combination of these fundamental causes. Genetics clearly play a role in disease. However, genes never operate in isolation from the environment. Environmental effects explain why observed differences in health disparity by socially defined race are greatly in excess of genetic differences between groups, in many cases in the wrong direction. The mechanisms associated with diseases of homeostasis, lack of maintenance, and by-products of defense systems, as well as those arising from stochastic developmental problems and maternal–paternal and maternal–offspring fitness conflicts, evolved very early in our species and are thus shared by all human populations. However, all are profoundly influenced by evolutionary mismatch, that is, the mismatch between the environments of our present circumstances and those in which are ancestors evolved. In the pages that follow, I argue that the greatest perturbation of human environments is that caused by social hierarchy. In the specific case of racial health disparity, it is the toxic environment generated by racial injustice.[58] I will illustrate this in detail in chapters that address aging and the lifespan, hypertension, cancer, and infectious disease. I will also describe how our microbiomes and the mechanisms of gene expression in the epigenome are affected by racial injustice. And I will demonstrate that a sharp distinction exists between the evolutionary (and holistic) understanding of health disparity and the racialist understanding of health disparity that currently dominates both biomedical research and clinical practice.

Chapter Two

DON'T BLAME IT ON PANDORA

The ancient Greeks called the first woman Pandora. She was created by Hephaestus on the order of Zeus. Her name in Greek loosely translated means "bringer of gifts." Yet she is remembered not for her benign gifts to humanity but for her curiosity, which led her to release all the evils upon the world. This happened when she opened a jar (also called "Pandora' box") filled with various evils including pestilence and death. The connection between Pandora and the Judeo-Christian Eve is apparent. Indeed, biblical scholars suggest that the Hebrew story may have been derived from the earlier Greek story about Pandora. Also because of her curiosity, Eve is tempted by Satan in the form of a serpent to eat the fruit of the forbidden tree of knowledge, which she shares with Adam. For this transgression against God's commandment, both are cursed. Eve is told that her pain in childbirth will be greatly increased and that her husband will rule over her. Adam is told that by the sweat of his brow, he will eat his food until he returns to the dust that he was created from.[1] The curse was generational.

The idea that sickness and death resulted from divine curses was not universal. Many Native American peoples accepted these as aspects of the circle of life. People were of the earth, and they returned to it. Thus, sickness arose when people were out of balance with the earth. For some West African peoples, death was just part of the beginning. For the Fulani people, the god Doondari first created worry, but when worry became too proud, he created death, which defeated worry. Others thought that death was the creator, Sa, who was present at the beginning of the world and played an essential role in creating it.[2]

Supernatural creation narratives tell us little about how living things work. In some cases, they are informed by the observations that ancient people made about nature. For example, "Let the earth bring forth creatures after their kind," attributed to J, one of the authors of Genesis, was an accurate observation of what people had seen with their own eyes, though J didn't describe the order of creation accurately. According to this tale, it was humans first, then plants, but we know that this is incorrect because no humans existed when the first microbial forms of life evolved on this planet about 3.5 billion years ago. However, creation narratives provide a unique insight into the societies and cultures that produced them. The fact that Pandora and Eve were held responsible for sickness and death coming into the world speaks to the patriarchy of the ancient Greeks and Hebrews. Eve's story is revealing in its singling out of two essential evolutionary adaptations of our species: intelligence and the difficulty of childbirth. In the Garden of Eden narrative, Adam and Eve lived complacent lives in obedience to the commands of God. Their sin involved eating from the tree of knowledge, which could be interpreted as an illustration of their desire to think for themselves. Yet, this narrative fails logically in that it does not explain why a supreme being would create an organism with a highly developed brain but then command that organism not to use it. Our offspring have large heads that house large hominid brains. This is what causes the pain in childbirth experienced by human females. Large head size conflicts with the earlier human adaptation of standing upright, which altered the skeletal architecture of the pelvic girdle. Our closet living evolutionary relatives, chimpanzees, do not experience childbirth pain because chimpanzees have a much smaller ratio of head size to pelvic girdle than do humans.

The garden narrative also fails by presenting a false notion of the relationship of humans to nature. The Garden of Eden was created to meet all the comfort and nutritional needs of Adam and Eve. Yet we know that plants do not "naturally" provide nutrition for animals. Plants are living organisms whose characteristics evolved to ensure the propagation of their own species, not to feed herbivores (plant-eating animals). The plants that humans now rely on for food are the product of thousands of years of conscious selection. Ironically, by producing these plants, humans created the conditions for the spread of a new suite of diseases that carry with them an extended period of sickness that eventually leads to our deaths.[3]

GOD DID NOT CURSE AFRICANS

Our species first evolved in Africa.[4] If this was because of the action of a supreme being, we are left to question why that being would make the first sapient beings inferior to those who would evolve later. Or, if you have no need for a supreme being in this narrative, you can ask why the first modern humans that evolved on this planet would be inferior to those who evolved later. The correct answer to both questions is that African populations are not inferior to any other branches of humanity. Therefore, to understand why some of us die sooner than others, we need to understand why any of us die at all.

Some sorts of death are easier to understand than others. When our ancestors first evolved on the plains of East Africa, we were prey to many species, including leopards and lions. These species are still dangerous, but more humans in Africa are now killed by hippos and crocodiles than by large cats. At the other end of the scale, humans die from parasitic infections caused by a bewildering variety of microbes (e.g., viruses, bacteria, single-celled eukaryotes, parasitic worms). We were recently reminded of our vulnerability to infectious organisms during the COVID-19 pandemic. However, in large part because of modern technology, far fewer deaths were caused by COVID-19 than by the great influenza pandemic of 1919, which some estimates say resulted in more than one hundred million deaths wordwide.[5] In addition, people have always died from accidents, droughts, starvation, and war, what are referred to as external (or extrinsic) causes of mortality. In the context of the evolutionary classification of disease presented in chapter 1, these are environmental sources of illness and death.

In the story of Oedipus, the Greek Goddess Hera sends the sphinx (a monster with the head of person and the body of a lion) to plague the people of Thebes. The sphinx sits atop a mountain overlooking the city and poses a riddle to anyone wanting to leave. If one fails to provide the correct answer, the sphinx devours that person. The riddle goes as follows: "What has four legs in the morning, two at noon, and three in the evening?" The sphinx was referring to development, adulthood, and senescence (aging).

The author of this myth was simply describing what people had observed about the life course. Humans are born unable to walk and thus crawl on all fours; they then learn to walk on two legs and do so for most of their lives; finally, they grow old and become infirm, requiring a cane. Ancient mythology and philosophy had no explanation for aging other than as a supernatural curse. Medieval scholars could not explain it. Nor could the early participants of the scientific revolution of the sixteenth century, such as Francis Bacon. In the main, it was taken for granted that all living things aged. In the nineteenth century, chemical theories were proposed suggesting that living things aged according to the general laws of thermodynamics. Of these, the second law seemed to have the greatest utility for explaining aging; it states that the disorder of the universe (entropy) always increases. This explains why an engineer will never be able to design a perpetual-motion machine. All machines must eventually break down through wear and tear. Living things, including humans, were understood the same way: we are simply biochemical machines that must eventually break down and cease functioning.

THE EVOLUTION OF AGING

Charles Darwin and Alfred Russel Wallace, the co-discoverers of evolution by natural selection, proposed that aging must be an evolved characteristic of living things. This realization was quite an act of intuition. Neither knew much about the microbial world. Nor did they understand that organisms such as bacteria that reproduce by symmetrical binary fission (one cell dividing into two identical daughter cells) do not age. This is because if a mutation occurred in a daughter cell that reduced its physiological function and caused senescence, the progeny of the impaired cell would not replicate its genome at the same rate as its sister lineage. The greater population size of the cells without the mutation would guarantee that they monopolized the resources of the environment. The lineage with the deleterious mutation would eventually go extinct.

August Weismann, the German cytogeneticist (a person who studies inheritance by looking at cell structures), then recognized that the key to aging must be associated with the fact that multicellular organisms evolved a division of labor between cells that produce gametes (germ cells found in the ovaries and testes) and those that carry out the necessary actions for the organism's survival (somatic cells, which compose the rest of the organism). Put simply, the central rule of biology is that "a chicken is simply an egg's way of making another egg." Thus, in every species and every generation, the key is to transmit as many copies of one's genetic code into the next generation as possible. As this occurs in environments that are not constant, successful living things evolve new tools to carry out this biological necessity as needed. If you take this dictum to its logical conclusion, you will understand that all humans currently alive are descended from the first living things, which biologists collectively call the last universal common ancestor (LUCA).

Your immediate ancestors were humans not so different from yourself. You probably knew your grandparents and may have been lucky enough to have known your great-grandparents. The number of your ancestors doubles each generation into your genetic past. Thus, you have two biological parents, four biological grandparents, eight biological great-grandparents, and so on. If you have Eurasian ancestry, you are descended from people who first entered that region of the world about fifty thousand years ago. However, those Eurasians were descended from people who had left Africa in a series of migrations that began roughly between two hundred thousand and one hundred thousand years ago.[6] As so little genetic change occurred during our migratory expansion, this means that every human on the planet is still essentially African. Differences relate only to when and how our ancestors left Africa. At some point, your ancestors were not modern humans; before that, they were not primates; and before that, they were not even mammals. If you keep going back, your ancestors were not even multicellular organisms. This is why all living organisms on Earth share some genes in common, and pretty much all living things use DNA as their genetic code and the same coding dictionary to produce proteins from messenger RNA. At some point in the evolution of life, senescence evolved from organisms that reproduced by symmetrical binary fission.

The scientific study of aging did not begin in earnest until the twentieth century because until that time, no core unifying theory to explain biology existed. In the middle of the twentieth century, however, that theory arrived in the form of the neo-Darwinian synthesis. This term refers to the unification of the principles of natural selection and of the particulate genetics first worked out by Gregor Mendel in 1866. Darwin's theory of natural selection was formulated without a correct theory of inheritance, which Mendel was able to provide with his concept of the gene. Via a series of careful experiments, he showed that some traits were produced by inheritance factors that were dominant over others. For example, he crossed two strains of true-breeding peas, one with green fruit and the other with yellow fruit. The first generation of the cross produced plants that produced only green fruit. Yet when the first-generation hybrids were mated to one another, the ratio of plants producing green to yellow fruit was three to one. By these experiments,

Mendel demonstrated that there were underlying rules to inheritance and that the expected traits of offspring could therefore be predicted by the traits of their parents.

The significance of Mendel's work was not recognized right away. It was first published in German, resulting in its being ignored by the English-speaking world until the turn of the twentieth century. However, once its significance was appreciated, its applications became readily apparent. Most importantly for this story, mathematicians began to recognize how they could use Mendel's principles to explain how the frequencies of genes would be determined within populations that bred at random. They were also able to work out which factors had to be at play for population gene frequencies to deviate from the expected values if all genotypes within a population were equally likely to mate with one another. These problems attracted some of the greatest scientific minds of the twentieth century, including Ronald Aylmer Fisher, John Burdon Sanderson Haldane, Sewall Wright, Thomas Hunt Morgan, and Theodosius Dobzhansky. I am a direct product of that intellectual synthesis, which allowed me to participate in helping solve one of the greatest problems in the history of biology: why organisms age.[7]

The chicken-and-egg metaphor explains how aging evolved. To bring this metaphor home to my students, I usually conduct a thought experiment with them. I begin by revealing that I am a wizard with great magical powers. (If you have attended any of my lectures, you will have seen how the students unquestionably accept that claim.) I then snap my fingers and say that I have stopped all aging in their bodies; thus, their physiological capacities will never dim. In your mind's eye, you can probably see the gigantic smiles that come to their faces. I follow this up with a question: "If we hold a class reunion one hundred years from now, how many of you would be alive to attend?" Most take the bait and say, "All of us." But there are always a couple more deeply thinking students who say, "Not all of us." They recognize that I said that I could cure their aging but that I did not say that they would be immune to other—extrinsic—causes of death like accidents, infectious diseases, and murder (predation). Thus, even without aging, they would all eventually die. Now imagine that instead of students, we are talking about a species of chicken. This species has evolved perfect physiological mechanisms to prevent age-related deterioration but at the cost of losing the ability to make eggs. This species would also eventually go extinct. This thought experiment makes the point that natural selection would never allow an organism to produce grandiose physiology at the cost of reproduction. Indeed, it is the opposite: reproduction is the name of the game. The amount of reproduction varies across species, but how long an organism lives is in reality an "afterthought" of the evolutionary process. What natural selection hones is the capacity to grow to adulthood and produce offspring. Thus, our somatic bodies are just the means by which our germ material (our genes) is passed on to the next generation. Life on this planet could not have evolved any other way.

THE EVOLUTIONARY THEORY OF AGING

In his book *The Genetical Theory of Natural Selection*, first published in 1931, Ronald Fisher shared a critical mathematical idea that allowed subsequent scientists to work out how aging could evolve. He derived an expression for an organism's reproductive value (R_0) and showed that this value was related to the stages of the organism's life cycle. For biologists, these stages can be divided into conception through first reproduction (development), the reproductively active period (adulthood), and postreproduction (senescence) (see figure 1.3). The organism's evolutionary fitness (defined as its reproductive success) during development is zero; during adulthood, it is greater than zero; and during senescence, it is again zero. The power of natural selection to remove genes that negatively affect this process from a population is strongest during development and strong during adulthood but declines toward zero as an organism nears the end of its reproductive period. You might ask why natural selection would allow the evolution of mechanisms that keep organisms alive when their future reproductive value is zero. The answer is that it does not. Many organisms do not have a postreproductive lifespan. Mayflies complete their entire life cycle in about twenty-four hours; the last day of life for female fruit flies grown in a laboratory is the day they lay their last egg; male salmon die off after they have mated. And most mammals do not have an appreciable postreproductive lifespan.[8] Why the great apes, including humans, have prolonged postreproductive lifespans is an active area of research (and a topic for another book).

In 1952, the British biologist Peter Medawar wrote a book titled *An Unsolved Problem in Biology* that expanded on Fisher's idea of the reproductive value. Medawar reasoned that if a "genetical disaster" occurred late enough in life, then natural selection would have no capacity to remove the bad gene from the population. If true, this would mean that species can accumulate genes as long as their age-specific negative impacts on fitness occur after the reproductive value (R_0) goes back to zero, that is, in senescence. Medawar eventually won a Nobel Prize for his work in immunology, but I would argue that his thinking concerning the inability of natural selection to remove alleles that contribute to aging was his most important contribution to science.

Shortly after the publication of Medawar's work, another great theorist of evolutionary biology, George C. Williams, proposed a second mechanism that could allow genes that contribute to aging to accumulate in populations. Williams reasoned that any gene whose impact on fitness in early life (development and adulthood) was beneficial would increase in the population despite its effects in later life, even if those effects were negative. He called this phenomenon "antagonistic pleiotropy."[9] The term *pleiotropy* refers to a gene whose product is involved in multiple physiological pathways and therefore influences several physical traits at the same time. Think of it like a switch that, when flipped up, causes several banks of lights to turn on at the same time and, when flipped down, causes those banks of light to turn off at the same time. The *antagonistic* in *antagonistic pleiotropy* refers to the fact that a gene may be "good" under one set of conditions but "bad" under another. In this case, the gene is good in early life but bad in late life. Put simply, the genes responsible for bringing you into existence are also the ones responsible for ending your life.

The mechanisms put forward by Medawar and Williams in the 1950s made possible a comprehensive theory explaining how aging could evolve. From 1960 to 1980, improvements were made to the theory. However, theories are just theories until someone tests them. Albert Einstein's(1879–1955) eloquent theory of space and time, the general theory of relativity, published in 1915, uses the metaphor of a tightly stretched piece of fabric for the three-dimensional nature of space and time: if you were to place a massive enough object on the piece of fabric, it would pull the space and time in its vicinity downward. The theory predicted that space and time would curve near massive objects such as stars and black holes. This was a neat idea, but it couldn't be accepted as true until someone could figure out a way to test its predictions. One crucial test of the prediction that light would be deflected near the sun was performed by Arthur Eddington and his collaborators in 1919. During a total eclipse, Eddington and other astronomers trained their telescopes on the sun and showed that light had indeed "bent" in its vicinity.

The critical test of the evolutionary theory of aging occurred in the mid-1980s. As with the quest to determine the correct structure of the DNA molecule, several laboratories were engaged in designing experiments to demonstrate that aging evolved and was determined by the interaction of the genetic mechanisms of mutation accumulation and antagonistic pleiotropy. The first two laboratories to conduct these seminal experiments were the Luckinbill laboratory at Wayne State University in Detroit, Michigan, and the Rose laboratory at the University of California, Irvine. (I am the only scientist to have worked in both laboratories: Luckinbill for my PhD and Rose for my postdoctoral research.)[10]

The results of these experiments were published in the journal *Evolution* in September 1984.[11] The authors demonstrated that the timing of an organism's reproduction determines its lifespan. Both the Luckinbill and Rose teams altered the schedule of reproduction in fruit fly populations. The control populations had their eggs collected to found the next generation at around two weeks. These flies could have continued reproducing, but they were killed by the researchers, so their lifespan from egg to adult was two weeks. Whereas the experimental groups had their egg collection schedules increased across generations, in the Rose laboratory, the experimental group had their eggs collected at ten weeks, and in the Luckinbill laboratory, the eggs were collected at about eight weeks. Thus, the flies in the experimental groups had to have genes that allowed them to survive to eight or ten weeks and be capable of reproducing at that age. Antagonistic pleiotropy was demonstrated by the fact that the flies in the control groups had superior early-life reproduction but shorter lifespans (genes good early, bad late) than those in the experimental groups, whereas the files in the experimental groups had lower early-life reproduction but longer lifespans (genes bad early, good late). Subsequent experiments (some of which I designed and participated in) demonstrated mutation accumulation in these flies.[12]

The results of these experiments explained how lifespan and the process of aging occur in all multicellular species, including fungi, plants, and animals. The genetic mechanisms of aging that were validated in flies operate in all these forms of life. Additional experiments with other fruit fly species, roundworms, yeast, and plants found the same essential results. This meant that the evolutionary theory of aging could now be used to make sense of the wide variety of lifespans found in multicellular eukaryotes. For example, a clone of a quaking Aspen tree in Utah named Pando has been aged at 990,000 years, a Great Basin bristlecone pine in the White Mountains of California at 4,856 years, fungal mushroom fairy rings at more than 3,000 years, and lake sturgeon at more than 120 years. The secret to the very long lifespans of these organisms does not result from their cell structures because they all share the same fundamental components. In the case of these organisms, their reproductive fitness increases with their size. Thus, for organisms like this, natural selection favors genes that allow the organisms to survive for a long period of time, letting them grow larger and thus produce more offspring.

Unfortunately, for a number of practical reasons, we could not repeat these experiments on the evolution of aging in mammals. The first is simply the cost. In the 1990s, the cost of maintaining a single laboratory mouse was about six dollars per day. To get data equivalent to that of the fruit fly experiments would have required populations sizes of about one thousand mice per selection treatment, and each selection treatment would have needed at least three to five populations. In addition, because of the longer lifespan of mice, the duration of the experiments would have to have been much longer than those conducted in fruit flies and roundworms.

However, the fly and worm experiments illustrated an important proof of principle, specifically the existence of a genetic trade-off between survivorship and reproduction—as would be predicted by antagonistic pleiotropy. And it turns out that you can mimic the effects of natural selection on this trade-off by altering the caloric content of mammals' diets. It had long been known that many rodent females will devour their offspring under starvation conditions. This behavior makes sense in that under these conditions the young would not survive anyway. Thus, by returning the caloric content of the young to herself, the mother increases the probability that she will survive until food is abundant enough to reproduce again and ensure the survival of her offspring. The early caloric-restriction experiments in mice showed that if you fed them considerably fewer calories than they would normally consume (e.g., 20 percent less), their bodies would shut down reproduction, resulting in an increase in their lifespan relative to the control group, which had been allowed to eat as much food as they wanted. These experiments demonstrated that caloric restriction could increase lifespan in rodents by about 50 percent. Further, the calorie-restricted rodents were found to have a decreased risk of cancer and type 2 diabetes, as well as neurodegenerative, autoimmune, and cardiovascular disease.[13] Experiments using fruit flies found the same.[14]

THE GENOMICS OF AGING

Over the last thirty years, our understanding of the genomic foundations of aging has increasing dramatically. Much of this work was conducted by researchers working with fruit flies, particularly Michael Rose and his collaborators. Advances were greatly accelerated by the advent of next-generation sequencing (NGS) technology, which enabled the "omics" revolution of the early twenty-first century.[15] "Omics" refers to the totality of specific factors within a cell, tissue, or organism. It is concerned with the characterization and quantification of entire sets of biomolecule structure, function, and dynamics. NGS greatly reduced the time needed to read the sequences of DNA (genomics), RNA (transcriptomics), and protein molecules (proteomics). Imagine that you are a detective called in to investigate a murder that occurred at a party. Genomics tells you who was at the party; transcriptomics tells you what each guest was doing at the party, and proteomics tells you which guests were most likely to have been involved in the murder.

In the early days of our experiments of the evolutionary theory of aging using fruit flies, we used the tools of classical genetics to estimate how many genes were involved in controlling aging. The estimates were not particularly informative, ranging from just a few to almost all genes! But in the early years of the twenty-first century, researchers began using the tool of two-dimensional protein electrophoresis to try to answer the question. In a study of the Rose laboratory fly populations, scientists were able to estimate that about 2 percent of the fly genome—about two hundred to four hundred genes—was responsible for the differences in lifespan they observed between short- and long-lived populations.[16]

With the advent of NGS, more accurate estimates of the genetic influences on the lifespan of these flies was possible. The genome of the fruit fly *Drosophila melanogaster* consists of 180 million base pairs. To put this in perspective, the bacterium *E. coli* has a genome of about 4.6 million base pairs, the plant mustard weed about 125 million, and humans about 3.3 billion. By the way, the size of an organism's genome does not correlate with its organizational complexity; for example, the bacterium *E. coli* has 6,000 protein-coding genes, the fruit fly has 13,937, the mustard weed has 27,416, and a human has 20,364.[17]

In 2017, my collaborators and I published a paper that examined the contribution of single-nucleotide polymorphisms (SNPs) (single changes to the DNA code); insertions or deletions to the DNA code (small insertions or deletions of nucleotides; i.e., the insertion or deletion of a C, T, A, or G); and transposable genetic-element (TGE) insertions (called "jumping genes," TGE insertions are insertions of larger segments of DNA that have the capacity to move and insert themselves at random places in the genome during DNA replication).[18] Any change in the DNA code has the potential to cause disease; for example, the sickle cell anemia is caused by a single-nucleotide change in the gene that encodes the hemoglobin B protein. Alternatively, single-nucleotide changes can be beneficial, such as the one associated with lactase persistence in the lactase gene. Because the lactase gene shuts down in all mammals once an infant is weened, this mutation was beneficial for human populations that domesticated cows and drank their milk past weening.

It should be apparent that insertions and deletions to the DNA code tend to be bad and that big insertions, like those caused by transposable genetic elements, can be really bad. However, there are cases of TGE insertions being beneficial, including one that occurred in the ancestor of jawed fishes about five hundred million years ago. This insertion helped produce the capacity to generate diverse antibodies against infection, which allowed the further development of an adaptive immunity system observed in all tetrapod vertebrates, including mammals. Our adaptive immunity relies on this ancient TGE insertion.[19]

In our NGS fruit fly study, we found that only sixty-four SNPs (in a genome of 180 million base pairs) were strongly differentiated between the short-lived flies (two-week generation) and a longer-lived fly line (four-week generation). However, our estimate was really an underestimate because we had used an extremely restrictive definition of a statistically significant difference. In this kind of study, called genome-wide association (GWAS), the standard probability value used to determine statistically significant difference is one in one hundred million ($p < 10^{-8}$), but we used $p < 10^{-180}$. We did this because, unlike most clinical studies using GWAS, we were able to rigorously control the environments in which the flies were grown, and we knew that we had imposed a particular regime of laboratory artificial selection. Yet even under these rigorous conditions, in one comparison between an extremely short-lived line and the longer-lived line, more than ten thousand SNPs met the $p < 10^{-180}$ criterion. We also found a difference in the number of TGEs associated with the lifespan of the short- versus longer-lived flies (about 340 versus about 211, respectively).

NGS methods have also allowed the examination of the population genetic mechanisms of aging in humans. Evidence suggests that the

TABLE 2.1
Population genetic mechanisms consistent with the evolution of aging

Mechanism	Early life	Late life	Examples
Mutation–selection balance	–	–, 0, +	Cat eye syndrome results from an inverted duplication at chromosome position 22q11. This variant cannot contribute to senescence because natural selection prevents the frequency of such variants from rising above the mutation rate.
Mutation accumulation	0	–	Hundreds to thousands of variants are associated with cataracts, diabetes, and osteoporosis, as well as cardiovascular, gastrointestinal, immunological, musculoskeletal, neurological, and respiratory diseases.
Antagonistic pleiotropy	+	–	ABCG8 and ABCG5 are associated with high cholesterol, lipid-related diseases, gallbladder disease, and cholelithiasis; ADH1B is associated with cardiovascular disease and gout; and SLC39A8 is associated with osteoarthritis.

Note: Variants may have negative (−), neutral (0), or positive (+) effects on evolutionary fitness.

The population genetic mechanisms associated with aging: mutation accumulation and antagonistic pleiotropy. Variants may have negative (−), neutral (0), or positive (+) effects on evolutionary fitness.

Sources: H. M. Dönertaş et al., "Common Genetic Associations Between Age-Related Diseases," *Nature Aging* 1, no. 4 (2021): 400–412; E. Long and J. Zhang, "Evidence for the Role of Selection for Reproductively Advantageous Alleles in Human Aging," *Science Advances* 9, no. 49 (2023): eadh4990.

mutation accumulation mechanism influences aging in humans. A recent study examining disease progression using data from the UK Biobank found that genetic variation associated with many diseases (cataracts, diabetes, and osteoporosis, as well as cardiovascular, gastrointestinal, immunological, musculoskeletal, neurological, and respiratory diseases) aligned with the mutation accumulation mechanism (table 2.1).[20] The diversity of age-related diseases associated with mutation accumulation is unsurprising simply because of the sheer number of genetic variants in the human genome that do not negatively affect reproductive fitness in early life. The impact of these neutral early-life variants differs by population, however, since their frequency is determined by genetic drift. Thus, as mentioned in chapter 1, a study of mutation accumulation variants associated with late-life disease in a European population might not replicate entirely for African or Asian populations.

The antagonistic pleiotropy mechanism also operates in humans. For example, one study used genomic data to test the relationship between reproduction and lifespan via data from the death registry of 276,406 UK Biobank participants.[21] This study showed a strong negative genetic correlation between variants that increased reproductive traits versus those that increased lifespan. This means that individuals with greater reproductive output had shorter lifespans than those who had less. Those with more genetic variants associated with higher reproduction displayed lower survivorship to age seventy-six years. This was also demonstrated when the researchers examined individual genetic variants associated with reproductive success. They found that the antagonistically pleiotropic variants discovered in this analysis were most often associated with cis-regulatory effects across multiple tissues or on multiple target genes (as would be expected for this mechanism). A study using data from the UK Biobank and the 1000 Genomes Project also demonstrated the existence of SNPs whose frequency was driven by antagonistic pleiotropy. They found that loci *ABCG8* and *ABCG5* showed antagonistic pleiotropy with high cholesterol, lipid-related diseases, gallbladder disease, and cholelithiasis (the formation of gallstones); *ADH1B* showed antagonistic pleiotropy with cardiovascular disease and gout; and *SLC39A8* showed antagonistic pleiotropy osteoarthritis.[22] This study thus showed that diseases common during human aging are produced by the action of genes that were beneficial during early life.

A notable omission of this study is that it chose not to examine the genes associated with cancer. Contrary to popular belief, cancer is not a single disease. Rather, it is a group of diseases characterized by uncontrolled cell growth. Cancer is also intimately related with aging, as shown in figure 2.1. In figure 2.1, the death rate per 100,000 people shows that the increase in cancer mortality begins to rise exponentially after age fifty; figure 2.2 shows that the age-specific birth rate of US women drops to approximately zero at age fifty. The correlation here is predicted by Fisher and Medawar's idea that any "genetical disaster" that occurs after net future reproduction is zero will not be acted on by natural selection. Thus, in the case of cancer, there is an excellent reason to suppose that the frequency of cancer-predisposing alleles is driven by antagonistic pleiotropy: because most cancers arise in stem cells. Stem cells play a vital role in the maintenance of tissues in multicellular organisms. They replace cells in tissues such as bone marrow and in the epithelia of the lungs, gut, and skin. In addition, the embryonic stem

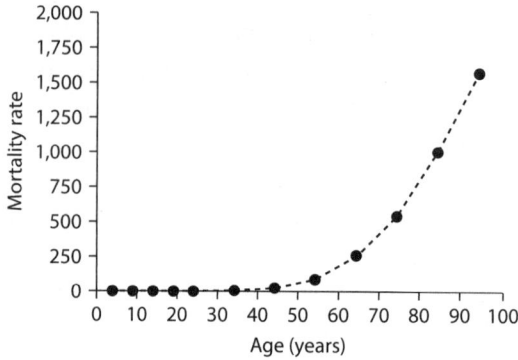

FIGURE 2.1. Age-specific death rate from cancer, 2019. During the development and reproductive periods, there is little cancer mortality. The inflection point (change in slope) for cancer mortality begins between 40 and 50 years of age. After this age the rate of mortality increases exponentially. (Data from *National Vital Statistics* 70, no. 9 [2021].)

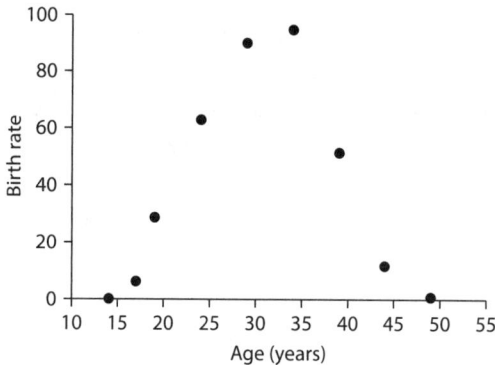

FIGURE 2.2. Birth rate per 1,000 women by age, United States, 2020. The birth rate has dropped to near zero by age 50; this is the same age range in which the increase in cancer mortality begins. (Data is births per 1,000 women, *National Vital Statistics* 70, no. 17 [2022].)

cells of placental mammals' invasive placentas contain much of the genetic program needed to produce cancer. Thus, fewer mutations are required in such stem cells to result in their loss of control of cell division, and thus these traits that are advantageous to an organism in early life (during development and adulthood) are deleterious in late life.[23]

This phenomenon can be observed in the gene mutations that increase the risk of ovarian and breast cancer, *BRCA1* and *BRCA2*. For example, one study showed that women of European descent with these mutations living under conditions of natural fertility (i.e., they were born before 1930) had more children, shorter interbirth intervals, a later age of last birth (beneficial to early-life reproductive success), and higher postreproductive mortality (detrimental to late-life survival) than did women without the mutations.[24] Several other cancer-related genes have also been shown to increase early-life fitness, including *AR*, *TP53*, *PTPN11*. *BRCA1* and *BRCA2* are tumor-suppressor genes with allele frequencies that differ by population. It is hard to know what the actual frequencies of these alleles are because not all breast cancers are caused by variation in the *BRCA1* and *BRCA2* genes and the medical literature generally reports frequencies by known cases of breast cancer cases as opposed to all members of a population. However, we do know that the allelic variants that cause early-onset breast cancer are rarer than those with later onset.

The increase in prevalence of the *BRCA1* and *BRCA2* genes in the Ashkenazi Jewish population has been linked to the drastic reduction of this population in Eastern Europe in the Holocaust of World War II. In this population, about 2 percent of individuals now carry *BRCA1* or *BRCA2* allelic variants associated with breast cancer, a frequency much higher than in non-Jewish people of Eastern European descent.[25] Studies of the *TP53* gene also show that the frequency of individual variants varies by population. One study examined variation in five cancer-associated genes (*BRCA1*, *BRCA2*, *KRAS*, *TP53*, and *PTEN*) in 681 healthy Americans.[26] In this study, 51 percent of participants were male, 49 percent were female, and the average age was forty-nine years. Results were grouped by the participants' recent ancestry as determined by genomic sequencing. Ancestries included African, African European, Central Asian, East Asian, European, Hispanic, and other. You may be confused deciphering these categories because they do not match the five socially defined races used by the US Census Bureau (white, Black, American Indian/Alaska Native, Asian, and Pacific Islander). The reason for this incongruence is that both researchers and the Census Bureau try to fit continuous human genetic variation into neat categories. As the criteria being used to make the categories are arbitrary, there is no reason for the categories to consistently classify individuals. I explain why this doesn't work in *Racism, Not Race*, a book I coauthored with Alan Goodman.[27]

In the study of five cancer-related genes, Africans, East Asians, Central Asians, and Europeans were defined by more than 80 percent of their genome displaying a recent signature from those regions (the remaining 20 percent could be from anywhere else); African Europeans were defined as having 20 to 90 percent European ancestry and 20 to 80 percent African ancestry (suggesting that for many in this category, one parent was primarily of European descent and one was primarily of African descent); and Hispanics were defined as having a "tri-ancestry" of African, European, and Native American origins (at varying percentages owing to the complex recent history of colonialism in the Western Hemisphere). The "other" group represented those whose genome signatures did not fit easily into any of the other categories. Consistent with other studies of global genetic variation, Africans showed the highest average number of cancer gene variants per individuals (84), followed by African Europeans (75.6, midway between Africans and Europeans), Central Asians (71.6), East Asians (68.6), Hispanics (68.3), and Europeans (64.5). The range of distribution of the number of cancer variants overlapped for all groups, meaning that any person from any group could have had a number of cancer-associated variants higher than the mean of another group. However, most importantly, this study used biomolecular modeling to predict how "dangerous" each cancer-associated variant was likely to be and found the groups to have the following number of dangerous variants per person: Central Asians, 2.2; Africans, 2.1; African Europeans, 2.0; Hispanics, 1.9; East Asians, 1.8; and Europeans, 1.8. In short, the genetic contribution to cancer from these five genes is roughly equal for people of these ancestry groups. Suggesting the idea that there is a simple genetic explanation for differences in cancer prevalence and mortality across socially defined racial groups is simply not tenable.

This study also suggested that about 40 percent of its cohort of 681 individuals would die of cancer. However, it has been observed that virtually all humans who live to advanced age have various cancers active in their somatic tissue at the time of death. Thus, cancer may not be recorded as the cause of death but may have been a significant contributor. The leading cause of death in the United States is currently heart disease. But this was not so in the early twentieth century, nor was it true of human populations in our ancient past. Diseases such as cancer, stroke, and heart disease are called "diseases of civilization" and reflect a dramatic change in how humans have come to live: from the hunter-gatherer environments in which we evolved to the agricultural and industrialized modern societies of the present day.

EXCEPT IN THE LIGHT OF EVOLUTION

Shortly before his death, the great evolutionary geneticist Theodosius Dobzhansky said that "nothing in biology makes sense, except in the light of evolution."[28] Over the course of the twentieth century, a bewildering number of theoretical developments and experiments examining nearly every arena of biological study have demonstrated the truth of this dictum. However, medicine has been incredibly refractory to the results of evolutionary science. This fact is even more startling when one considers that the most challenging phenomenon faced by medicine in the twentieth century was the rapid spread of antibiotic resistance in microbes and the emergence of new viral pathogens in humans. The only way to understand these phenomena was to use evolutionary biology.

Progress in communicating the significance of evolution to medicine began with the 1994 publication of the book *Why We Get Sick: The New Science of Darwinian Medicine* by the psychiatrist Randolph Nesse and the evolutionary biologist George C. Williams.[29] The strength of Nesse and Williams's analysis stimulated others in the fields of biological anthropology, evolutionary biology, biomedical research, and clinical medicine to begin to use evolutionary reasoning to understand why disease exists. This has led to a better understanding of fundamental underlying causes and thus to the development of new approaches to treatment. One example of this is fever, an adaptation that evolved to raise the body's temperature above levels that allow successful replication of bacteria and viruses. Thus, one should treat fever only when the temperature is approaching the point that the risk of damage to critical systems (such as the brain) outweighs the beneficial effect of controlling pathogens. And coughing is an evolved adaptation to expel infectious pathogens from the lungs; as with fever, treatment should be given only when risk of damage outweighs benefit. Antibiotics and antivirals should not be taken to completely irradicate infection. Evolutionary models demonstrate that antibiotics should be used to drive pathogen levels to a point at which the host's immunity can control the infection. Attempting to irradicate microbes always fails and in fact spurs the rapid evolution of antimicrobial resistance.

You should now recognize that we cannot blame the existence of disease and death in our species on supernatural curses. Pandora and Eve are innocent. Disease and death exist because we are evolved entities whose sole biological purpose is to replicate our genomes into the next generation.

However, in the pages that follow, I will demonstrate that there is no genetic reason for any socially defined racial group to suffer from disease and death more than another. On average, we should all make our threescore and ten. Indeed, progress in modern biomedical research—when united with the evolutionary theory of aging—has the potential to greatly improve both health and lifespans. At least for those who can afford the treatments.[30]

Geographically based genetic variation exists in our species, and some of it plays a role in predisposing individuals to particular patterns of disease and death. However, the magnitude of that genetic variation cannot explain the appalling differences in health profiles that we observe in industrially advanced societies. Indeed, in *The Race Myth*, I titled the chapter on health disparities "America Is Enough to Make You Sick," channeling the words my mother used to say to me when I got on her "last nerve" during my adolescence. I watched my mother and so many relatives and friends experience lives of pain and premature death owing to the combined forces of structural racism and poverty. In the pages that follow, I will explode the myth of the "genetically sick" African and call to account a society that refuses to face the facts and lacks the political will to enact the promise of its founders: "liberty and justice for all."

Chapter Three

THERE IS NO SLAVERY GENE

Debunking the Myths of Hypertension

In chapter 1, I mentioned that hypertension is one of the diseases resulting from a dysregulation of homeostasis. Remember that because homeostatic mechanisms must be plastic and adjustable, they are vulnerable to being locked into maladaptive states. Similar to other diseases of homeostasis, a predisposition to hypertension is made worse by novel environments; this is referred to as evolutionary mismatch. Recent work has demonstrated that rates of hypertension are increasing dramatically across the world. One culprit for this is the mass introduction of salty and highly processed foods into the modern diet. In industrialized nations, this is augmented with the availability of these foods in great excess of people's caloric needs. This in turn causes the dysregulation of an evolved defense mechanism associated with osmoregulation (salt balance). The combination of these factors, along with other environmental factors differentially experienced by Black and Brown people, explains the patterns of hypertension we see in our racially structured society. West and Central African populations were not historically predisposed to hypertension, nor did natural selection for salt retention result in the survivors of slavery being predisposed to hypertension in the Americas.

BLACK PEOPLE HAVE HIGH BLOOD PRESSURE

Virtually everyone in my extended biological family has suffered from or is currently experiencing high blood pressure. Hypertension is defined as systolic pressure higher than 140 and a diastolic pressure less than 90. Systolic pressure is the pressure measured when the heart is contracting, and diastolic pressure is the pressure measured in the arteries when the heart is relaxed between contractions. Hypertension is associated with an elevated risk of stroke, cardiovascular disease, heart failure, and renal (kidney) failure. Hypertension can both cause these conditions and be the result of these conditions.

Since the 1930s, American physicians have believed that people of African descent are innately prone to hypertension. Hypertension was also observed in Afro-Caribbean populations beginning in the 1960s.[1] In 2015–2016, uncontrolled hypertension by socially defined race and ethnicity in the United States was reported as follows: non-Hispanic Black, 40.3 percent; Hispanic, 27.8 percent; non-Hispanic white, 27.8 percent; and non-Hispanic Asian, 25.0 percent.[2] Rates of controlled hypertension (hypertension controlled by medication) were as follows: non-Hispanic white, 50.8 percent; Hispanic, 45.0 percent; non-Hispanic Black, 44.6 percent; and non-Hispanic Asian, 37.4 percent. These figures mean that more non-Hispanic Black people have hypertension, but fewer are getting treated for it.

Hypertension is not just a problem in the United States. More than 1.4 billion people worldwide have it. The greatest burden of hypertension is experienced in low-to-middle-income countries, where 75 percent of the global total reside.[3] The prevalence of uncontrolled hypertension in sub-Saharan African countries ranges from 15 to 70 percent, the wide range resulting partly from differences in the characteristics of those sampled, particularly age.[4] Thus, hypertension is a disease of not only homeostasis but also maintenance. In a sample of more than 110,000 sub-Saharan Africans, the prevalence of hypertension by age was as follows: age thirty, 16 percent; age forty, 26 percent; age fifty, 35 percent; and age 60, 44 percent.[5] A similar age-related increase also exists in the United States, with more than 40 percent of Americans having hypertension.[6] Hypertension rates are also rising across the globe, even in children, as a result of evolutionary mismatch associated with the introduction of ultra-processed foods to the modern diet.[7] However, it is thought that the age-associated increase in blood pressure occurs only in industrialized nations, not in hunter-gatherer groups such as the

Khoi-San with a "normal" salt intake.[8] For example, a recent study found that the overall rate of untreated hypertension in Nigeria was 29 percent (about the same as in non-Hispanic whites in the United States).[9] An awareness of the prevalence of hypertension in Nigerian populations is important for understanding the potential genetic roots of blood pressure variation in African Americans owing to the role that that region played in supplying people for the transatlantic slave trade.[10] Further, hypertension is not just a problem in Africans. For example, a recent study of untreated hypertension in a population from Southern Iran reported a prevalence of 46.6 percent (about the same as non-Hispanic Blacks in the United States).[11] According to the 1997 US Office of Management and Budget categories used in the US census, Iranians would be classified as white; however, the census categories released in 2024 now include the category of Middle Eastern and North Africans. A study of hypertension in Iranian immigrants to the United States from 2002 to 2011 found that they had lower rates of hypertension than did those living in Iran in 2019.[12] This story underscores that we cannot assign simple racialized genetic causality to blood pressure differences among human populations.

BLOOD PRESSURE IS A QUANTITATIVE GENETIC TRAIT

A person's blood pressure is determined by cardiac output and resistance to blood flow in the peripheral circulation.[13] Cardiac output in turn is determined by blood volume (which is influenced by the amounts of sodium, mineralocorticoids, and atrial natriuretic peptide in the blood) and cardiac factors (heart rate, contractility). Resistance in the peripheral circulation is determined by factors in bodily fluids such as hormones and other molecules that constrict the blood vessels (angiotensin II, catecholamines, thromboxane, leukotrienes, and endothelin). Conversely, other hormones and molecules dilate the blood vessels (prostaglandins, kinins, and nitrous oxide). Neural factors such as constrictors (alpha-adrenergic) and dilators (beta-adrenergic) and local factors (autoregulation, pH, hypoxia) also affect resistance in the peripheral circulation.

The heritability (i.e., the degree that children are similar to their parents in a particular trait) of blood pressure is thought to range from 0.30 to 0.50. Heritability estimates are always contingent on the populations used to make the estimates and the environmental conditions under which the traits were measured. Therefore, these estimates will always be variable. The estimate I report here resulted from the use of genome-wide association (GWAS) methods. The study that produced these estimates concluded that 1,477 single-nucleotide variants (SNPs) accounted for 27 percent of the estimated heritability of blood pressure. This means that other genetic variants, as yet unidentified, account for the remaining 73 percent. Further, the variants identified in this study are also known to affect other traits in addition to blood pressure; this is an example of pleiotropy (i.e., genetic variants that influence multiple physical traits). You will recall from chapter 2 that antagonistic pleiotropy plays a major role in determining the lifespan of multicellular organisms. The variants identified as influencing blood pressure are also statistically associated with variation in body fat levels, alcohol intake, birth weight, height, heart rate, blood cell type distribution, educational attainment, and socioeconomic status. All these traits are also influenced by environmental factors, both physical and social, further complicating how blood pressure variation will manifest in any group living under variable environmental conditions.

Finally, because most GWAS studies have been conducted on European and East Asian populations, we cannot be sure that African populations display the same range of heritability as Eurasians or that these estimates are the same in African Americans. Remember that African Americans have on average 16 percent European genetic ancestry.[14] One study attempted to test whether SNPs found to contribute to hypertension in European Americans also contributed to hypertension in African Americans.[15] The results of this study must be taken with a large grain of salt (no joke intended) because the sample size was only 9,534 individuals, which is substantially underpowered to find statistically significant variants by modern GWAS standards (which often require hundreds of thousands to one million participants). The study examined the impact of fourteen variants associated with hypertension risk in European populations on African Americans. Of these, only five were shown to have a statistically significant impact on lowering or raising systolic or diastolic blood pressure or on hypertension risk.

Table 3.1 shows the frequency of some of these variants in African and European Americans, their odds ratios, and the probability of computing those odds ratios by chance alone. Some SNPs with a positive odds ratio increase the risk of higher systolic pressure, higher diastolic pressure, or

TABLE 3.1

Frequency of SNPs associated with hypertension risk in African Americans and European Americans

Nearest gene	SNP	Trait	Frequency, African American	Frequency, European American	Odds ratio	P value	Group
CASZ1	rs880315	Hypertension	0.17	0.34	1.14	3.35×10^{-3}	All
CASZ1	rs880315	Hypertension	0.17	0.34	1.13	0.03	> 30 to 60
RSPO3	rs1361831	Diastolic pressure	0.13	0.46	−1.96	0.02	> 60
CDH13	rs30996277	Hypertension	0.33	0.21	1.26	1.5×10^{-3}	> 60
PLEKHG1	rs17080093	Systolic/diastolic pressure	0.22	0.08	−2.99/−1.69	0.02/0.04	< 30
C10 or f07	Rs1530440	Systolic/diastolic pressure	0.03	0.19	4.16/2.57	0.04/0.04	< 30

hypertension, and SNPs with a negative odds ratio decrease these risks. In this study, African Americans were found to have higher frequencies of two SNPs that decrease risk and lower frequencies of four SNPs that increase risk. European Americans were found to have higher frequencies of one SNP that lowers risk and higher frequencies of four SNPs that raises risk. This means that, on average, African Americans have a genotype that is *more* protective against hypertension than that of European Americans. However, this study does not provide the whole genetic picture for hypertension as many loci are involved, which, owing to the different linkage relationships of Africans and Europeans, would not be found by this technique. That said, the results provide little support for the notion that genetics alone are responsible for most of the disparity in hypertension rates between African and European Americans.

A "JUST SO" STORY OF HYPERTENSION

Stephen Jay Gould (1941–2002), a preeminent evolutionary biologist of the late twentieth century, was fond of debunking adaptationist explanations of evolutionary biology concepts in the style of the "Just So" tales of the English author (and white supremacist) Rudyard Kipling. You might remember stories such as "How the Leopard Got His Spots" or "How the Camel Got His Hump." These and other of Kipling's stories relied on the reader accepting every claim because each claim built the next. If one rejected any claim in the narrative, the story collapsed like a house of cards. Adaptationist narratives operated in the same way. This approach viewed every aspect of the organism as having arisen from natural selection, and it downplayed the role of chance forces in evolution, such as genetic drift, and the impact of the environment on physical traits.

The "slavery hypertension" hypothesis is a "just so" story that was promulgated in the twentieth century.[16] It began by proposing that before the transatlantic slave trade, West and Central Africa lacked a salt supply. The authors of the slavery hypertension hypothesis further reasoned that survival during the warehousing, transport (via the Middle Passage), and acclimation of Africans into slavery was facilitated by greater salt retention. An additional explanation for the higher prevalence of hypertension in African Americans was supplied in the early 1990s; it associated hypertension with the hormone norepinephrine, a by-product of melanin production during times of stress. It was thus argued that more Black people had hypertension than white people because they had more melanin and experienced more stress than white people.

However, the slavery hypertension hypothesis had several fatal flaws, including the fact that West and Central Africa had no shortage of salt at the time of the slave trade. In addition, records of mortality during slave voyages indicate that there were many causes of death unrelated to salt retention. Therefore, it is highly unlikely that a strong natural selection for salt retention existed in enslaved African people.[17] One could just as easily argue that people of Northwest European ancestry adapting to the subtropical conditions of the Western Hemisphere should have undergone strong selection for sodium retention to resist heat exhaustion—but that theory never appeared in the biomedical literature.

METABOLIC SYNDROME

Metabolic syndrome is a disease associated with hypertension.[18] This condition is characterized by a dysregulation of glucose (sugar) metabolism. It is defined by central obesity (based on population-specific criteria) and any two of the following: increased triglycerides, reduced high-density lipoprotein (HDL) cholesterol, increased blood pressure, and increased fasting glucose or diagnosed diabetes).[19] As with many complex diseases, metabolic syndrome shows great disparities by socially defined race.[20] In 1960, 1.8 percent of the US population had diagnosed type 2 diabetes, but by 2018–2019, more than 11 percent had the condition. Further, metabolic syndrome appears in racially subordinated populations at a rate almost twice that of socially dominant populations.[21]

GWAS studies have identified more than four hundred genomic variants associated with increased risk of type 2 diabetes.[22] Geneticists can use the number of genomic variants associated with elevated risk that a person has to compute what is known as their polygenic risk score (PGS). Put simply, the more of these variants that you have in your genome, the higher your risk. However, a person's PGS for type 2 diabetes accounts for only about 10 percent of its heritability in groups that are predominantly European in ancestry.[23] Clinical measurements adjusted for age, sex, and parental diabetes—such as body mass index, systolic blood pressure, fasting glucose, HDL cholesterol, and triglyceride levels—have performed better than PGS in predicting the occurrence of type 2 diabetes.[24] However, socially defined race is often heavily implicated in differences in the prevalence of type 2 diabetes. The dominant narrative of biomedical research overemphasizes the differential frequency of genomic variants associated with type 2 diabetes while underemphasizing environmental influences, some of which are associated with structural racism.

ENVIRONMENTAL CAUSES OF HYPERTENSION

The GWAS study discussed in the previous section established that 65 to 85 percent of the risk of developing hypertension is caused by the environment, with only 15 to 35 percent contributed by an individual's genotype. The one great truth of the American experience is that its socially defined races have always been differentially affected by environmental factors. In 1587, English colonizers established a settlement on Roanoke Island in what is now North Carolina; by 1590, the colony had ceased to exist. Most colonizers likely starved to death or succumbed to disease after being weakened by poor nutrition, but some may have joined (by choice or force) the Croatoan people, the descendants of whom have a much higher frequency of the blue-eye allele than would be expected by chance alone.[25] Within a century, the dynamics of colonization changed. The massive influx of Europeans—and the Africans they had enslaved—led to the disruption of the environments of Indigenous people. Indigenous people were exposed to pathogens for which they had no resistance, and epidemics of smallpox and other infectious diseases decimated their populations along the Eastern seaboard.[26] This, in conjunction with the physical violence deployed by Europeans against them, which resulted in the seizure of their lands, led to their lower survivorship and reproduction under colonialism.

Social subordination almost always results in a combination of lower levels of survivorship, reproduction, and well-being in the subordinated. In chapter 1, I mentioned that fragmentary evidence showed that the lifespans of enslaved people were significantly lower than those of their enslavers. In *The Emperor's New Clothes* (2001), I described patterns of age-specific survivorship for African Americans relative to European Americans surviving into the late twentieth century. In *Racism, Not Race* (2022), Alan Goodman and I showed that this pattern is still with us in the twenty-first century. And in a widely read paper that I published in 2023, we discussed how this pattern of social subordination invariably results in reductions in well-being among racialized individuals.[27] Interestingly, the impact of social subordination on survivorship is not limited to humans. It is observed in all social species.[28]

Numerous components of our modern environment contribute to the escalating rates of hypertension and associated diseases globally. You don't have to be a biological scientist to figure out most of the contributing factors, which include diet (e.g., an excess of food, ultra-processed foods, high salt content, high sugar content), toxic metals (e.g., lead), endocrine-disrupting chemicals, poverty, lack of education, excessive workload, trouble sleeping, continuous tension, annoyance, and emotional stress.[29] For example, certain environmental elements that many people take for granted, such as green spaces, have a profound effect on hypertension risk. Such factors are differentially distributed by socially defined race, as is proximity to a toxic waste site. In this regard, socially defined race is a much more powerful predictor of location relative to toxic waste than is social class.[30] The degree to which any American is exposed to the risk factors associated with hypertension is determined by a combination of identity factors associated with social status, including wealth, education, socially defined race, ethnicity, occupation, social class, gender, and sexual orientation. With regard to a given disease context, these variables have different weights. However, together, they are far more powerful predictors of hypertension and associated sickness and mortality than are the minor genetic differences we observe among socially defined races.[31] For example, collectively, these factors continue to explain disparities in mortality from heart disease between Blacks and whites (see figure 8.1).

This pattern of environmental effects, which drives health disparities in the form of structural racism, is the central theme of this book. It is found over and over in the disease systems I will discuss. However, this reality is often lost on medical practitioners because most medical textbooks, particularly in pathology, do not address the social determinants of health. Instead, disparities in even the rarest of diseases are claimed to be associated with some genetically based disparity in molecular or cellular physiology. This is the thorniest of the misconceptions that must be overturned in biomedical research and clinical practice—and that is what I hope to accomplish in this book.

Chapter Four

RACE AND THE MICROBIOME

The vast majority of living things on this planet are microbes. Microbes can be divided into two main types: viruses that do not conduct cellular metabolism and are therefore obligate parasites and organisms that conduct their own metabolism. In the taxonomic classification of living things, organisms with a metabolism are classified into three domains based on their cellular organization: Bacteria, Archaea, and Eukarya. This classification arranges groups hierarchically by shared attributes, which are ultimately encoded in their genes. As an example, table 4.1 provides the levels of classification for *E. coli* and *Homo sapiens*.

The number of bacterial species is estimated to be greater than one billion, and there must be many more viral species than species that conduct their own metabolism.[1] For example, 219 viral species are known to be capable of infecting humans.[2] Although we do not know how many viral species there are, it is estimated that there are ten nonillion (10^{30}) viral particles on the planet—more than the number of stars in the known universe. Single-celled microbes were the first life forms to evolve on Earth about 3.5 billion years ago, long before the first multicellular macroscopic organisms came into existence about one billion years ago. Biologists before the nineteenth century paid them little heed because the tools to study them did not exist. Yet none of us would be here without these microbes because they play essential roles in the biogeochemical cycles of elements such as carbon, nitrogen, sulfur, and phosphorus. They also inhabit the bodies of multicellular

TABLE 4.1
Classification of living things: Bacteria and Eukarya

Domain	Bacteria	Eukarya
Kingdom	Eubacteria	Animalia
Phylum	Proteobacteria	Chordata
Class	Gammaproteobacteria	Mammalia
Order	Enterobacteriales	Primates
Family	Enterobacteriaceae	Hominidae
Genus	*Escherichia*	*Homo*
Species	*Coli*	*sapiens*

Note: The levels of biological classification are based on shared features. In Bacteria, the definition of species is more fluid because gene-sharing between species identified by physical and metabolic characteristics is common. In Eukarya, the species definition is based on the ability to share genes during sexual reproduction.

organisms. The estimated number of microbes normally associated with the human body is between ten and one hundred trillion![3] Compare that to the average number of cells that make up the adult human body: thirty-six trillion for men and twenty-eight trillion for women.[4] Microbes inhabit our skin, nasal passageways, gut, and even brain. Most are commensal (feeding on or in our bodies but causing no harm); some are symbiotic (conferring essential molecules to our bodies, such as vitamins); and a few are pathogenic. Even normally commensal microbes can become pathogenic under certain circumstances. The "normal" microbes of the human microbiome also prevent the colonization of pathogenic microbes.

THE MICROBIOME RESEARCH RACE

Research on the potential health impacts of the microbiome is relatively new. A recent review article on the significance of microbiome research to public health cited no sources published before 2011.[5] However, the work was born into an existing scientific enterprise complete with historical shortcomings related to socially defined race. As human microbiome studies are in their infancy, we really know very little about the relationship of microbial community taxonomic composition and functional characteristics and how these are associated with human biological variation.[6] What we seem to know is that the microbiomes of any individual vary over time and in conjunction with the phases of life (i.e., infancy, adolescence, adulthood, and senescence). However, a great deal of individual variation exists in the composition of microbiomes, even in people of good health and supposedly the same ancestry. Further, knowing the species composition of a microbial community does not always tell you how the community functions. This is because bacteria have particularly high levels of horizontal gene transfer. This means that individuals within the same species (or between species) can share genes by means of self-replicating segments of DNA known as plasmids. The plasmids with the highest rate of transfer between individuals and species are often those that carry genes for antibiotic and heavy metal resistance, often both.[7] This results in a great diversity of function in bacteria that are members of the same species or genus. For example, only about one-third of the genes in the gut microbiomes of healthy individuals have been found in all people tested.[8] Therefore, it is possible that microbial communities of somewhat different taxonomic composition can be functionally equivalent. We still have no comprehensive sampling of human microbiome diversity that would allow for a correlation between geographically based human genetic variation and microbiome composition. In the absence of such data, attempts to racialize the human microbiome seem to result from the preexisting assumptions of researchers about the significance of biological race and ethnicity in determining the biological attributes of people.

However, some general patterns have emerged concerning the microbiome diversity of people living in industrialized nations versus those living in less industrialized and thus what could be considered more traditional ways of life. These differences are most likely the result of factors such as antibiotic use, diet, food preparation, culture, and industrial pollution, as well as the presence of heavy metals and novel chemicals affecting the microbes found in industrialized nations. At least one study has shown a rapid shift in the gut microbiome of people migrating from underdeveloped to industrialized countries to match that of individuals in the destination country.[9]

SOCIALLY DEFINED RACE, MICROBIOMES, AND HEALTH DISPARITIES

Microbiome studies have not been free from the assumption that socially defined race should be a determinant of microbiome composition. Of course, many researchers who hold this view operate under the false assumption that socially defined races actually represent legitimate biological units within our species. An excellent example of the "inherent racial" assumption is provided by a study of the skin microbiome communities of Chinese individuals published in the journal *Science Reports*.[10] The study examined the composition of the skin microbiomes of two hundred people living in Hong Kong and compared them with publicly available datasets from the rest of China, Tanzania, and the United States. While one can understand why the researchers chose to compare their samples with samples from the rest of China, there was no logical reason to compare them with samples from Tanzania or the United States. It is hard to comprehend what hypothesis they were testing.

In the Hong Kong sample, the researchers found 52 phyla, 137 classes, and 750 genera. Of these, bacteria within the phyla Actinobacteria (36.6 percent), Proteobacteria (31.6 percent), Firmicutes (19.1 percent), and Bacteroidetes (7.1 percent) made up more than 94 percent of the organisms in the samples. They also found a one-thousand-fold difference in skin community composition by individual and that factors such as household location, age, ventilation, and site from which the skin sample was taken were significant in determining the diversity of the microbiome sample. Using statistical analysis, the researchers were able to differentiate the total microbiome samples by location (i.e., China, Hong Kong, Tanzania, and the United States), as well as by the site from which the samples were taken, such as the palm, forearm, and forehead. This study thus demonstrates that microbiome variation within an individual is actually much greater than the variation between the four population groups being compared.

The evidence that false racial assumptions underlay this study is in its title: "Skin Microbial Communities of Chinese Individuals Differ from Other Racial Groups." The paper's design illustrates the typological thinking of the authors, reviewers, and editors. Given that the paper was published, all those involved must have believed that Chinese, Tanzanians, and Americans are different racial groups. Further, the United States is a nation whose socially defined racial and ethnic composition includes people from all over the world. Nowhere in the paper do the authors acknowledge how the ancestral diversity of Americans would have affected their analysis. It is likely that the authors viewed Americans primarily as people of European descent or that the database they used to make their comparisons was composed primarily of samples taken from people of European descent. This is not an unreasonable assumption about most of the biomedical data in US data repositories.[11]

Even more interesting is that the authors' statistical analysis was able to differentiate the skin samples of people from Hong Kong from those of people from the rest of China. I am unaware of any racial typology that differentiates the residents of Hong Kong as a separate biological race from people living in the rest of China. Further, the researchers' own analysis indicated that skin microbiome composition was influenced by many variables that had nothing to do with host genomic composition, variables that were clearly differentiated between groups in the societies being compared (Tanzania and the United States). For example, altitude and exposure to ultraviolet (UV) light, particularly UV-B, have been shown to influence skin microbiome composition.[12] UV-B has a wavelength of 280 to 315 nanometers (nm), while UV-A has a wavelength of 315 to 400 nm. The energy of light waves is inversely proportional to their wavelength, so UV-A exposure actually causes less damage than UV-B exposure. UV-A is associated more with skin wrinkling, whereas UV-B is associated with skin cancers such as malignant melanoma. UV exposure is directly related to latitude. The continental United States is north of the Tropic of Cancer and lies roughly between 35°N and 48°N, whereas Tanzania is in the tropics and situated at about 1°S to 12°S. So, any skin microbiome composition differences observed between these groups is more likely to result from differences in sunlight exposure than from any genetically determined differences in the skin itself.

A recent study by Brooks et al. attempted to differentiate gut microbiomes across "ethnicity" in the United States.[13] The study examined gut microbiota from 1,673 individuals of self-described ethnicity from the American Gut Project and the Human Microbiome Project. Four groups were compared: Caucasians (N = 1,237), Asian-Pacific Islanders (N = 88), Hispanics (N = 37), and African Americans (N = 13). Individual microbiome data was classified by self-reporting, meaning that the participants self-described their race and ethnicity. The researchers then grouped them into four categories. The problem with this classification scheme as a means to evaluate biological processes is obvious. For example, the social category of Asian-Pacific Islander includes a large swath of human biological diversity extending from Eurasia to Melanesia. The Hispanic category is equally troublesome as this population is defined by language, not biological ancestry: Puerto Ricans have on average 72 percent European, 16 percent Amerindian, and 12 percent African ancestry, whereas Mexican Americans have on average 46 percent European, 51 percent Amerindian, and 3 percent African ancestry.[14] The term *Caucasian* is often used to refer to people of European descent but does not describe where in Europe these individuals' ancestors came from. Further, *Caucasian* is a nineteenth-century anthropological term that also includes people from North Africa, the Middle East, and the Indian subcontinent. However, the authors used the term only to describe people who would be socially classified as white in the United States. There is also variation in the African American category, where the average percentage of European ancestry ranges, on average, from 16 percent to more than 30 percent in states such as West Virginia and Washington. Thus, the largest difficulty with the classification scheme used in this analysis is that it conflates biological race with social conceptions of race, as well as with ethnicity. *Ethnicity* refers to shared national, cultural, and linguistic origins, whereas *socially defined race* incorporates an arbitrary mixture of social and cultural characteristics along with biological ancestry. Neither scheme is useful for testing the basis of any sort of biological variation—unless that variation is in a *biological* outcome that is the result of differential exposure to *sociological* variables.

Brooks et al. found that individual variation in gut heterogeneity predominated, but the authors also claimed to have identified statistically significant degrees of total microbiota distinguishability for ethnicity, body mass index, and sex. They tested for ethnicity signatures in the gut microbiota using alpha and beta diversity, abundance and ubiquity distributions, distinguishability, and classification accuracy. Alpha diversity is the observed number of taxonomic groups or the evenness of their distribution, whereas beta diversity is the variability of the community composition across samples. For example, if one sample had fifty genera and the second had one hundred genera, the second would have higher alpha diversity. If one sample had four genera evenly represented (0.25, 0.25, 0.25, and 0.25) and the second had four genera unevenly represented (0.10, 0.10, 0.10, and 0.70), the first would have higher alpha diversity by the evenness criterion. In the case of beta diversity, if in ten samples the percentage of one taxon, such as Actinobacteria, was consistently 10 percent with a variance of zero and the second group of ten samples had a range of Actinobacteria percentages (10, 5, 50, 20, 30, 90, 70, 0, 80, and 20 percent) with a sample variance computed as 0.107, the second group would have greater beta diversity.

Brooks et al. found that the Shannon alpha diversity index (which weighs microbial community richness by number of observed operational taxonomic units [OTUs] and evenness) varied significantly across ethnicities in the American Gut Project dataset. An OTU can refer to an individual, species, genus, or family. OTUs are used in microbiome studies because taxonomic units are identified by the use of the DNA sequence of the 16S gene, which encodes the RNA of the small subunit of the bacterial ribosome, an essential structure involved in assembling all of an organism's proteins. Therefore, natural selection acts strongly against any changes in this sequence. Thus, this sequence is an excellent tool to measure the genetic relatedness of organisms because change in it is very slow. For example, the 16S sequences of the bacterium *E. coli* and all of the genus *Shigella* species are virtually identical.

The Shannon alpha diversity index rank (evenness, species number) used in this study was as follows: Hispanics > Caucasians > Asian-Pacific Islanders > African Americans. This meant that Hispanics had the most diverse, and African Americans the least diverse gut microbiome community. Given the issues with this arbitrary racial and ethnic classification mentioned earlier, it is unsurprising that the alpha diversity ranking was not consistent with prior studies; for example, the Human Microbiome Project sampled showed Hispanic = Caucasian > African American > Asian-Pacific Islander. However, the simple fact that there were only thirty-seven Hispanic and thirteen African American samples immediately invalidated the ability of this study to make claims about racial or ethnic variation in the microbiome. This is because it is impossible for such small samples to be representative of an entire population's microbiome composition. For example, in the 2020 US census, more than forty-six million people identified as African American. With thirteen samples, not even one African American per state was represented nor even one for the twenty states with the highest African American populations. Thus, while it is possible that the study's analysis could show statistically significant differences between the samples used in the analysis, the results would be meaningful only if the samples were representative of the distribution of microbiome variation in the larger populations from which they were derived. For example, if all the microbiome samples for Hispanics came from Puerto Rico, it is highly unlikely that they would represent all Hispanics living in the United States.

Another study illustrates how sample dependent the observations in the study by Brooks et al. were. This study, on the effect of stress on gut microbiome diversity, found no statistically significant differences between Black and white women.[15] The researchers compared the gut microbiota of forty-seven Black and thirty-three white women in Alabama, and they reported demographic and biological data. The mean body mass index and waist circumference of the Black women were found to be statistically significantly greater than those of the white women ($33.3 > 27.5$ and $98.3 > 86.6$, respectively). The diets of both groups were considered similar, but the white women reported statistically significantly greater life stress and greater distress events than did the Black women ($p = 0.026$, $p = 0.052$). In contrast to the greater life stress variable, the sample of white women sample consisted of more individuals with yearly incomes of more than $50,000 (seventeen white versus ten Black). The authors found no statistically significant differences in the alpha diversity of the gut microbiota of these groups (Shannon-Weaver diversity index: 5.19, 5.16; Simpson's diversity index: 0.93, 0.92).

However, the authors did find that Black women had greater beta diversity and abundance (more bacteria in the gut). As this study was interested in the role that gut biota play in predisposition to colon cancer, the researchers examined the abundance of seven taxa (genera) associated with the disease: *Bacteroides, Bifidobacterium, Clostridium, Fusobacterium, Lactobacillus, Porphyromonas,* and *Ruminococcus*. Of these, only *Bacteroides* had statistically significantly more abundance in the Black women sampled ($p = 0.035$). Each of these taxa plays an important role in our guts. *Bacteroides* breakdown oligo- and polysaccharides, providing nutrition and vitamins to us, as well as to other microbial residents. *Bifidobacterium* digest dietary fiber, also providing nutrition and vitamins. This group also helps prevent infection by pathogenic microbes. *Clostridium* plays a role in reducing inflammation and allergic responses. *Fusobacterium*, on the other hand, promotes inflammatory responses against pathogenic bacteria. *Lactobacillus* also plays a protective role by repairing damage caused by pathogenic bacteria such as *Clostridium difficile* and *Campylobacter jejuni*. *Ruminococcus* degrades complex polysaccharides, providing nutrients. The role of *Porphyromonas* in the gut is unclear. This study showed that the abundance of *Bifidobacterium* in the gut microbiome was associated with stress in both Black and white women. Thus, this study with slightly larger samples of Black and white women, whose ancestral and sociological attributes were better understood than in the study by Brooks et al., found quite different results. However, it should be recognized that neither of these studies examined enough people to be representative of the socially defined groups they were comparing.

A further study examined the gut microbiota of African American and "Caucasian" (European American) people from the Detroit metropolitan area of Michigan and found a dramatic difference in the community composition of these two groups.[16] The participants were being screened for colon cancer, all were male, the mean age of the African Americans was greater (65.2 years) than that of the European Americans (62.6 years); height was similar between groups (70.4 inches for the African Americans versus 69.0 inches for the European Americans); weight was higher in the European Americans (194 pounds versus 181 pounds); African Americans had more colon polyps (4.60 versus 1.43); and African Americans had more adenomas (noncancerous growths in the epithelial tissue) (3.8 versus 1.0). The bacterial genomic DNA of the participants was isolated from colonic effluents. In this study, 7,234 and 5,252 unique OTUs were found in the African American and European American samples, respectively, and just 742 OTUs were shared between groups. Alpha diversity was higher in the European American sample. Alpha diversity was calculated via the Shannon-Weaver index by sequences per sample; however, there was considerable overlap in the confidence intervals across sequences per sample. The European American samples showed twenty-four and African Americans only eleven phyla. The phylum level of classification is just below the kingdom level (e.g., Actinobacteria, Bacteriodetes). Of these, the African American and European American samples were 70.7 percent and 43.2 percent Bacteroidetes, and 22.8 percent and 36.2 percent Firmicutes, respectively. At the class level, there were more taxa in the European American samples beyond the major classes of Bacteroidia and Clostridia (about ten for European Americans versus six in African Americans). The study concluded that the percentage of proinflammatory species was higher in the African American samples than in the European American samples. This is important because systemic inflammation is associated with a variety of diseases including cancer. Dysregulated inflammation is another example of disease caused by a byproduct of defense.

The greater preponderance of proinflammatory species in the African American gut samples is consistent with the higher number of polyps and adenomas found in this group. Of course, this study doesn't tell us anything about why this disparity exists. Neither did the authors include samples from healthy participants (without polyps) to use as a control comparison. Thus, from this study, we really have no way of knowing whether the disproportionate numbers of proinflammatory taxa are responsible for the higher polyp count in African Americans. Nor do we know whether we would find the same differences in taxonomic distribution in healthier individuals from these socially defined groups. We also have no way of knowing how these differences in gut composition originated.

It is well established that dietary composition has powerful and long-lasting impacts on gut microbiota.[17] A study of the impact of dietary differences on gut microbiota conducted on children in Italy (Europeans) and Burkina Faso (Africans) showed that the latter group had less than half the Firmicutes composition (27.3 percent versus 63.7 percent) and twice the Bacteroidetes composition (57.7 percent versus 22.4 percent).[18] This difference in gut composition was shown to be associated with the differences in the diets of the two groups. The African children were eating a diet low in fat and animal protein but high in starch, fiber, and plant protein. The Italian children were eating a diet high in animal protein, fat, and sugar but low in fiber. A dietary difference of this sort between the African American and European American participants in the Detroit study could easily account for the pattern observed in these taxa—which is opposite to the one seen in the African and Italian children. It also highly likely that the lack of a difference in the gut taxa of the Black and white women in the Alabama study is associated with a greater similarity of African American and European American diets in the South than in the North. What is clear from these studies is that genetic variation between the groups involved does *not* drive differences in gut microbiome composition.

Exposure to UV-B light has been shown to affect the composition of the gut as well as the skin microbiome.[19] For example, a study showed that bacteria in the phylum Bacteroidota were in greater abundance in a sample of fair-skinned Canadian women described as Caucasian who lived at a latitude of 47°N compared with a sample of darker-skinned Yanomami Indigenous people living in South America at a latitude of 0°N to 4°N. Living at this latitude and generally wearing less clothing than those living in Canada mean that the Yanomami get greater sunlight exposure compared to Canadian women of European descent. This example illustrates that the composition of gut microbiota can be influenced by environmental factors that are not fully understood. Thus, findings of measured differences in gut microbiota composition between socially defined racial or ethnic groups must be interpreted with caution: do such differences result from some inherent ancestral and coevolutionary relationship with the groups in question or from differences in environmental exposures that the researchers are simply unaware of?

WHAT WE KNOW AND DON'T KNOW ABOUT RACE AND MICROBIOME COMPOSITION

Microbiome science is new. The tools for understanding microbiome diversity developed out of the principles of community ecology, most of which were established in macroscopic organisms. However, we know that there are vastly greater numbers and species of microbes than there are of macroscopic organisms.[20] In addition, microbes evolve and operate in their communities in ways that are not readily discernible from the biology of macroscopic organisms (e.g., horizontal gene transfer). The technologies that allowed the study of microbiome composition (e.g., DNA and RNA sequencing) also date to the late twentieth century. In reality, we are still working out how microbial communities assemble and how different environments affect their dynamics, especially those microbiome communities associated with multicellular organisms and how they influence the health of those multicellular organisms.[21]

Given that microbiome science is in its infancy, it is hard to understand why it has already been deployed as a tool to explain health disparities by socially defined race. Yet we know that the use of socially defined race as a descriptor of inherent biological difference is nothing new. It stems in part from the simple fact that most of those engaged in the scientific enterprise are people of European or East Asian descent who have never had to do any serious thinking about human biological variation and social definitions of race.[22] It also results from a lack of connection between the disciplinary training of many of the individuals now engaged in modern microbiome research (e.g., medicine, computer science, engineering) and the disciplines required to fully understand human biological diversity (e.g., anthropology, population genetics, quantitative genetics, evolutionary biology). An understanding of the latter disciplines is a prerequisite for recognizing the fallacy of typological racial schemes in nature, as well as the complexity of the genotype-to-phenotype pathway, especially in humans.[23] An individual's ability to maintain microbiome communities that positively contribute to their health is clearly a quantitative genetic trait (phenotype). As such, this phenotype results from the interaction of genetic and environmental factors, as well as the covariance of genes and environment.[24] The covariance of genes and environment refers to whether a specific genotype and environment are positively or negatively correlated with each other. I have argued that, because structural racism, the genes carried by African Americans are more likely to be associated with toxic environments.[25]

The fact that maintenance of what is considered a healthy microbiome is a quantitative genetic trait is evidenced by recent work estimating the heritability of gut microbiome composition.[26] This study examined 18,340 individuals from twenty-four groups (including African Americans, American Indian/Latin Americans, East Asians, Europeans, and Middle Easterners) and found that the gut microbiome composition of individuals was highly variable. The authors were able to identify a core microbiota, that is, a number of bacterial taxa present in more than 95 percent of individuals. It was composed of nine genera: *Bacteroides*, *Faecalibacterium*, *Blautia*, *Alistipes*, *Dorea*, *Roseburia*, *Subdoligranuium*, *Ruminococcus*, and *Lachnoclostridium*. Of these, the most abundant genus was *Bacteroides*, followed by *Faecalibacterium*, *Blautia*, and *Alistipes*. Using genome-wide association, the authors identified thirty-one genetic variants associated with gut microbiome composition ($p < 5 \times 10^{-8}$). However, these variants were not enough to calculate any heritability, meaning that an individual's genotype had virtually no impact on their gut microbiome composition. By extension, this demonstrates that population genetic differences between the included groups (which correspond to socially defined races in the United States) did not explain their microbiome composition either.

This is a powerful rejoinder to the attempts to use socially defined race as a biological category to explain the impact of the microbiome on health disparities. Yet we do know that an individual's microbiome composition can have powerful effects on their health profile. This is indicated by how the gut–brain axis is affected by microbiome composition.[27] It has been firmly established that there are bidirectional interactions among the brain, gut, and gut microbiome. Research has identified candidate signaling molecules with at least three communication channels. The communication in this system is complex, consisting of nonlinear, bidirectional pathways that contain multiple feedback loops, and it is likely that there are interactions between various channels. Alterations of gut–brain interactions have already been established for irritable bowel syndrome, but it is also likely that this system plays a role in psychiatric and neurological disorders.

Because socially defined race is intimately associated with various forms of subordination, racial groups do not share the same environments. Alterations in experienced environmental conditions undoubtedly affect the gut–brain system. This means that environmental and genetic influences and the covariance of genes and environment have had and continue to have major impacts on observed health outcomes, including those mediated by microbiomes. Finally, the misuse of racial concepts in microbiome research results from the fact that the scientific enterprise is intimately associated with the forces that wish to maintain the status quo of racism, colonialism, and capitalism.[28]

Microbiome studies attempting to address health disparities are also limited by their focus on taxonomic composition as to opposed to the function of the microbes. In actuality, what is far more important is the functional roles that various microbes play in specific communities and how these can be perturbed by various environmental inputs.[29] In an experimental study on zebrafish, feeding them copper nanoparticles or ionic copper sulfate at a concentration of 500 mg/kg dramatically disrupted their gut microbiomes.[30] Heavy metal pollution of water supplies is an issue faced by socially subordinated communities across the globe, and it has also been shown to disrupt our gut microbiomes.[31] In addition, lead in drinking water disproportionately affects pregnant mothers and children. For example, children absorb 40 to 50 percent of an oral dose of water-soluble lead compared to only 10 percent in adults.[32] Such lead absorption has been shown to have damaging lifelong impacts on developmental processes, in turn affecting intelligence, behavior, and achievement. Some of these impacts may result from microbiome dysbiosis. For example, in the city of Flint, Michigan, between 2013 and 2015, the amount of lead in children's blood increased from 2.4 percent to 4.9 percent owing to drinking water from an outdated water distribution infrastructure. In the most affected areas, the percentage was as high as 6.6 percent. The population of Flint is 70.6 percent African American, and in the areas that experienced the highest levels of lead, it is 78.8 percent African American.[33]

Clearly, any measurements of children's gut microbiome composition in Flint would have been affected by the amount of lead ingested. Flint is only one of the many examples of differential exposure to toxic environments that racialized people have faced in America since its founding. Thus, any evaluation of health-associated variables must be understood in this context. Further, any evaluations of genetic contributions to health-associated variables, including microbiomes, cannot be conducted because racially subordinated people have never shared the same environments as those with racial hegemony. Thus, as with other health-related variables, attempts to racialize microbiome differences on the basis of innate genetics are deeply flawed and harmful.

PART II

Harm

Chapter Five

INFECTIOUS DISEASE STRIKES UNEVENLY

The Poor Die More

Life on this planet has always been and will always be dominated by single-celled organisms. Most of these are free living; indeed, without their roles in biogeochemical cycles and the microbiome (see chapter 4), organisms like us could not exist.[1] However, many are parasitic, infecting the bodies of large-bodied multicellular organisms such as humans. In addition to the single-celled organisms with cellular metabolism, you can throw viruses into the parasitic mix. Because they do not have cellular metabolism, viruses are obligate parasites; they use the cellular machinery of living things to replicate their genomes. There are probably anywhere from one billion to one trillion bacterial species on Earth, and many more viruses.[2] And there are at least 1,513 bacterial species and at least 219 viral species that infect humans.[3] In addition to these, a large number of unicellular eukaryotes (organisms with cell structures like ours) also infect humans. They cause diseases such as skin and lung infections (various fungi), malaria (*Plasmodium*), sleeping sickness (*Trypanosoma*), meningitis (amoebas), and dysentery (amoebas). Finally, there are various flatworms (which cause diseases like schistosomiasis) and roundworms (such as *Necator*, which causes chronic anemia). With such a great diversity of microbes that want to eat us, it is amazing that our species has lasted as long as it has.

If we take a calendar year to represent the history of our planet, we have survived the equivalent of two minutes (in this imagining, we arrived on the scene on December 31 at 11:58 P.M.). However, bacteria and viruses have been here from the very beginning. The key adaptation that made organisms such as us possible is our innate and adaptive immune systems, which confer resistance against microbes. These evolved very early in animals, so we share elements of our innate immunity with organisms like jellyfish. Our adaptive immune system uses lymphocytes (white blood cells), which generate diverse receptors to identify pathogenic organisms via genetic recombination and somatic mutation. This system originated in the ancestors of the jawed fishes about five hundred million years ago (about November 9 in our calendar year analogy).[4] Despite how effective our adaptive immunity is, microbes always win in the end. Early in our lifespan, we're more capable of surviving acute infections, but this capacity declines as we age (as a consequence of lack of maintenance; see chapter 1). Microbes win because they evolve more rapidly than we do because of their short generation times and very large populations. This is why the human mortality rate from pathogens (e.g., COVID-19, respiratory syncytial virus, influenza) is always higher during aging than during our developmental and reproductive years.[5]

In chapter 1, you learned that pathogens are a common feature of the human environment. If that is so, why do some groups of people suffer more illness and death from pathogens than others? Specifically, what is it about structural racism in America that results in racialized people suffering more illness and dying more from infectious disease? In January 2020, the SARS-CoV-2 virus was first detected in the United States. Shortly thereafter, I participated in a series of interviews on the *Roland Martin Unfiltered* program.[6] In those early interviews, I warned that the virus would differentially affect Black and Brown communities across the United States. This was not because these groups were more genetically susceptible to the virus. As the virus had just crossed into humans from outside our species (bats or pangolins were the likely reservoir), no human population had greater innate immunity than any other.[7] I reasoned that the burden of sickness and death would be heavier on these people because the conditions of social life in these communities were more amenable to the transmission of an airborne virus. These conditions included crowding; poor ventilation; antiquated heating, ventilation, and air conditioning (HVAC) systems; a greater use of public transportation; the inability to stay home from work; and generally inferior access to health care.[8]

On July 5, 2020, *The New York Times* reported that the number of COVID-19 cases per one hundred thousand individuals in the United States for Whites, all groups, Blacks, and Latinos was twenty-three, thirty-eight, sixty-two, and seventy-three, respectively.[9] It has been shown that past racial discrimination played a powerful role in experiencing illness and death from COVID-19. In a study conducted between April and July 2020 in New York City, zip codes were used to study the likelihood of illness or death from COVID-19. It was demonstrated that neighborhoods with a higher proportion of Black and Hispanic residents had a higher percentage of infection. Historically redlined districts showed a higher likelihood of infection, even if they had recently been economically upgraded. This demonstrated that a preexisting social structure is still operating to influence health disparities.[10] The historical effect of redlining is a problem that my research group is currently investigating in the context of microbiome composition in the built environment experienced by residents in Greensboro and Durham, North Carolina.

Certain industries that employ disproportionate numbers of Black and Brown workers, such as meat packaging and processing, were required to continue operating during the pandemic. Many such employers discouraged workers from staying home if they were feeling ill, and some provided incentives to come to work during the initial phases of the pandemic. Unsurprisingly, these industries experienced high rates of COVID-19 infection and death.[11] Even worse was the fact that the Trump administration authorized the speedup of factory production lines during the early stages of the pandemic. This meant that lines were not only physically unsafe but also required workers to stand closer together than they normally would, thus increasing virus transmission.[12] Of course, this is the same administration that discouraged wearing masks, promoted pseudoscientific "cures," and held super-spreader events in the White House Rose Garden.[13] Ironically, it was Trump's attitudes that changed the racial profile of SARS-Cov-2 transmission in the following years. His followers were the least likely to get vaccinated. In September 2021, *The Washington Post* reported that the states with higher percentages of Trump voters in 2020, such as Florida, Kentucky, Mississippi, Texas, West Virginia, and Wyoming, had the lowest rates of vaccination and the highest rates of death from COVID-19.[14] More scholarly analysis demonstrated that in addition to Republican ideology, factors such as xenophobia, religiosity, trust in media, and trust in science also contributed to the higher prevalence and rate of death to this group.[15]

As of this writing, we now face another Trump administration whose grasp on the science of the prevention of viral transmission is questionable. In November 2024, President-Elect Donald Trump nominated Robert F.

Kennedy Jr. for the position of secretary of health and human services and David Weldon for the position of director of the Centers for Disease Control and Prevention (CDC).[16] Both are opposed to vaccination programs. In 2022, Kennedy's personal attorney lobbied the Food and Drug Administration for the abolition of childhood vaccination against polio.[17] Public health and research scientists circulated petitions calling for the senate not to approve Kennedy's nomination; however, with Republican control of the senate, he was confirmed. This could not come at a worse time given that recent evidence suggests that human-to-human transmission of H5N1 influenza (bird flu) may be on the horizon.[18] Should human-to-human transmission evolve, a rapid vaccine development program similar to the one that controlled the spread of COVID-19 will be necessary. Having a secretary of health and human services and a director of the CDC who oppose vaccines will not help make this possible.

THE RACIALIZATION OF COVID-19

While no population had any greater innate resistance to SARS-CoV-2, it was not long before attempts to racialize the severity of or resistance to the disease began to appear in the literature. This was unsurprising because, as mentioned, a belief in typological race concepts is still common among biomedical researchers and clinicians.[19] First and foremost, susceptibility to or resistance to any pathogen is determined by multiple genes, as well as environmental conditions. Thus, modern studies tend to use genome-wide association (GWAS) to evaluate these traits. For GWAS to give reliable results, large numbers of individuals are required. They are generally divided into two groups, one called "cases," consisting of people with the disease in question, and one called "controls," consisting of people without the disease. GWAS looks for specific loci associated with the disease at a probability higher than could be expected by chance alone. One of the earliest GWAS studies of severe COVID-19 infection examined 3,199 hospitalized individuals and 897,488 controls of non-African descent.[20] The researchers found that the most prominent risk variant was located between the *LZTFL1* and *CCR3* genes on chromosome 3. *LZTFL1* encodes the leucine zipper transcription factor-like 1, and *CCR3* encodes a chemokine. Chemokines control the migration of immune cells and positioning immune cells in our tissues. Thus, it is possible that both genes have something to do with susceptibility or resistance to viral infection. However, what is most note-worthy about this study is that it demonstrated that this risk variant most likely originated in Neanderthals. The Neanderthals (*Homo neanderthal-ensis*) are an extinct hominid species closely related to our species, *Homo sapiens*. The closeness of the two species was demonstrated by the fact that after *Homo sapiens* first left Africa between two hundred thousand and seventy-five thousand years ago, they began to interbreed with *Homo nean-derthalensis* across Eurasia and Southeast Asia.[21] This means that the risk variant for severe COVID-19 is not found in African populations. Indeed, this paper found that the frequency of the risk was lowest in European populations and then increased through Middle Eastern, Indian, Papua New Guinean, and Indigenous Australian populations. African Americans have small amounts of Neanderthal ancestry through their admixture with Europeans. Admixture occurs when offspring are produced by the mating of individuals from different geographical locations. For example, prior to Columbus's journey to the Western hemisphere, persons living in that por-tion of the world did not contain any recent ancestry from either Africa or Europe. However, shortly after this contact, mating between Europeans and Amerindians began, and soon after that Africans were added to these populations. Thus via this process of migration and mating, new admixed populations were produced; e.g., today's Mexicans are on average 51 percent Amerindian, 46 percent European, and 3 percent African ancestry; while Puerto Ricans are 16 percent Amerindian, 72 percent European, and 12 per-cent African ancestry; and finally African Americans are ~1 percent Amer-indian, 16 percent European, and 84 percent African ancestry.[22]

A later larger GWAS study differentiated COVID-19 infection into eight phenotypes. The researchers examined samples from more than 736,000 people using the AncestryDNA platform. Individuals were apportioned into the COVID-19 phenotypes via a questionnaire that determined whether they had had the virus, been hospitalized, been exposed but not tested posi-tive, and exposed and tested positive, as well as whether those who had been infected were symptomatic, paucisymptomatic (i.e., experiencing only a few symptoms or only mild symptoms), or asymptomatic, and how severe the disease was. The distribution of individuals by socially defined race and ethnicity was 73 percent European, 6 percent admixed Amerindian, 3 percent admixed African American, and 18 percent other. Sixty-seven percent were female. The study replicated twelve genetic variants that had previously been found to be associated with COVID-19 severity, including the locus inherited from Neanderthal ancestry (*SLC6A20/LZTFL1*, three single-nucleotide polymorphisms). The others were found in OAS3 (2'–5' oligoadenylate synthetase 3), *DPP9* (dipeptidyl peptidase 9), *IFNAR2* (interferon α and β receptor subunit 2), *TMPRSS2* (transmembrane serine protease 2), *STM2A* (alipoprotein E), *ABO* (α 1,3-N-acetylgalactosaminyl transferase and α 1–3 galactotransferase), *IGF1* (insulin-like growth factor 1), *CCHCR1* (coiled-coil α-helical rod protein), *KAT7* (lysine helical transferase 7).[23] Studies like this are limited in their capacity to undercover genetic variation associated with resistance or susceptibility to infectious disease because of the distribution of the participants, which was constrained by the data included in the AncestryDNA database. The vast majority of human genetic variation resides in African populations. Yet people of African descent composed only 3 percent of the study participants. As they were described as an admixed population, their African descent originated in West or Central Africa. But it is not clear from the methods reported in the paper how the researchers accounted for admixture. This is an issue because the linkage of genetic variants differs between sub-Saharan Africans and Europeans. Linkage blocks in the genome are smaller in African populations (because our species first evolved in Africa) and get larger with distance from Africa.[24]

The GWAS studies make it abundantly clear that you cannot racialize the genetic variation associated with resistance or susceptibility to COVID-19. Yet some studies presented exactly such a view of these traits. In 2020, a paper was published in the *Journal of the American Medical Association* (*JAMA*) examining racial and ethnic variation in the nasal gene expression of transmembrane serine protease 2 (*TMPRSS2*).[25] Previous studies had reported a differential expression of this gene between Black and white men and claimed that it was associated with a higher incidence of prostate cancer in Black men.[26] *TMPRSS2* is important in the penetration of SARS-CoV-2 into airway cells because the virus uses the protein it produces to initiate entry into those cells. This study used nasal epithelial cells collected from patients in the Mount Sinai Health System in New York City collected between 2015 and 2018. The authors extracted RNA (amounts of which are an indication of gene expression) and performed RNA sequencing. Nasal samples from 305 individuals were used, of which 8.2 percent were described as Asian, 15.4 percent Black, 26.6 percent Latino, 9.5 percent mixed race, and 40.3 percent white. Before discussing the results of this study, it is important to point out its limitations. First, this was a very small sample. There were only forty-seven Black people. Importantly, "Black" is a social definition, and the percentages of African and European ancestry in Black individuals varies widely. Further, the authors did not discuss the ancestry of the participants identified as Asian. How many had South Asian, Central Asian, East Asian, or Southeast Asian ancestry? How many were admixed with European ancestry? There was no description of the Latino population. Where they Caribbean or Mexican? What where their percentages of African, Amerindian, and European ancestry? None of these samples could be considered representative of their ancestral populations (a similar problem was identified with the study of gut microbiome diversity in chapter 4). These difficulties mean that no valid racial or ethnic conclusions can be drawn from this study, which raises the question of how it could have passed peer review as a study of supposed population diversity.

The study found a statistically different and higher expression of the *TMPRSS2* gene in the Black individuals compared with the other groups. This is not surprising since previous studies had also found a higher expression of this gene in Black people. Statistically significant differences in *TMPRSS2* expression were not found in the Asian, Latino, mixed, or white populations, but as a whole, these groups were statistically significantly different from the Black population. However, this differential expression does not mean that Blacks were somehow more vulnerable to SARS-CoV-2 infection than the other groups. The question that this study did not address was exactly how much expression (how much *TMPRSS2* protein on the surface of airway cells) was required to initiate successful entry of the virus into cells. The mean values reported in the paper for whites was 8.04 $\log_2$ counts per million, and for Blacks it was 8.64 $\log_2$ counts per million. This measure is a way of normalizing raw counts to account for sequencing depth. Taking the exponential of the $\log_2$ count results in the numbers 3,102 for whites and 5,653 for Blacks. If this is an estimate of the receptors available for SARS-CoV-2 infection, these numbers are much higher than what is required to initiate and maintain cell-to-cell infection. For example, HIV-1 requires only 3.2 proviruses to spread from cell to cell.[27] If the efficacy of SARS-Cov-2 infection is remotely similar to that of HIV-1, then the amount of the *TMPRSS2* protein available on the surfaces of nasal airway cells for viral entry for all groups was greatly in excess of that required to cause infection. Indeed, studies of SARS-Cov-2 transmission illustrate that very few viruses are required to successfully infect a cell.[28] Therefore, there is no reason to believe that the differences in gene expression found in the study had any impact on the differential infection rate observed in Black and Brown people in New York during the early days of the pandemic. In fact, early figures from that time showed that Latinos displayed higher rates of infection than Blacks despite the lower gene expression found in the Latino sample.

Further analysis of the role of *TMPRSS2* polymorphism demonstrated just how flawed the reasoning of the *JAMA* study was.[29] This study used bioinformatic methods to examine the distribution of genetic variants in two genes associated with SARS-CoV-2 susceptibility. Specifically, the researchers used an algorithm to survey the genomes in three databases for potentially deleterious nucleotide nonsynonymous substitutions. A deleterious non-synonymous substitution refers to a mutation that changes the encoding of a triplet code for an amino acid in a protein. If the substitution results in a protein that has impaired function, then we consider the substitution deleterious. The most famous example is the substitution in hemoglobin that causes sickle cell anemia. Here the functional protein has glutamic acid encoded by (GAG) at position 6 in the beta-globin, but the mutation changes the coding to (GUG) resulting in a valine amino acid. The result is a hemoglobin protein that causes red blood cells to sickle.

Returning to the study of SARS-CoV-2 susceptibility, in the angiotensin-converting enzyme 2 (*ACE2*) gene, they found sixty-three potentially deleterious allele variants, and they found that the distribution of these variants differed by population with a frequency of 0.39 and 0.54 in African Americans and European Americans, respectively. They found frequencies of 0.02 to 0.10 in the other populations surveyed (Latino/admixed American, East Asian, Finnish, and South Asian). Amish and Ashkenazi populations were also included, but they were found not to carry any of the variants. The authors found that the variants p.Met383Thr and p.Asp427Tyr, which have been reported to inhibit interaction between the SARS-CoV-2 spike protein and the ACE2 receptor protein in African populations, occurred at the very low frequencies of 0.003 and 0.01, respectively. These variants were not found in any other populations. From this fact, you would infer that African populations have slightly greater resistance to COVID-19 than the others in the study. The researchers found sixty-eight deleterious variants in *TMPRSS2*. Similar to *ACE2*, frequencies of 0.35 and 0.59 were found in African Americans and European Americans, respectively. The study made no particular associations between variation at this locus and susceptibility to COVID-19. The most important aspect of this study is that it examined a larger sample of genomes from more diverse populations than had been done previously. Its results suggest that there is no racial element to SARS-CoV-2 susceptibility; rather, all populations contained variants that might confer some resistance.

SAME STORY, DIFFERENT DAY

In the introduction, I described why and how the original association of American medicine with chattel slavery created the foundation for its typological beliefs about race. Both historical and bioarchaeological evidence demonstrates that enslaved people were differentially exposed to pathogens compared with their masters. This began during their capture and transport and continued once they were enslaved in the Western Hemisphere. Further, their conditions of social subordination made them more vulnerable to the diseases caused by those pathogens. These conditions included undernutrition, exhaustion from working very long hours, and the ongoing corporal punishment associated with slavery. Things were not much better for the few freed African Americans during the reign of chattel slavery. They were often underemployed, undernourished, exhausted from overwork, and psychologically traumatized from the constant fear of being kidnapped and returned to slavery, and they suffered from poor housing in free states. Mortality data suggest that they did better than their enslaved peers but less well than free whites. Bioarchaeological data on male skeletons suggest a higher rate of infection with flatworms and tuberculosis among free Blacks compared with whites.[30] Infant mortality for enslaved people was about twice that of free Blacks.[31]

The end of slavery did not greatly improve the situation. Lincoln's administration was not prepared to receive all the formerly enslaved people who escaped from plantations during the Civil War. Abolitionists such as Harriet Tubman did the best they could with limited resources to feed, house, clothe, and provide medical care for thousands of people classified as "contraband." African American men were often promised food and shelter for their families if they enlisted in the Union army, but in November 1864, the Union general Speed S. Fry broke his promise to these soldiers. He ordered his white soldiers to remove all freed people from a Union fortress, and the tent city that had been erected around the fortress was forcibly dismantled. This resulted in Black soldiers' families having no place to go for shelter or a reliable source of food.[32]

African American soldiers who fought for the Union were not protected from infectious disease. It is important to note that during the Civil War, disease accounted for more deaths than battlefield causalities. More than three-fifths of Union and two-thirds of Confederacy military deaths were caused by infectious disease.[33] The main culprits were pneumonia, typhoid, diarrhea and dysentery (caused by a variety of bacteria and protozoa), and malaria.[34] The main causes of death by infectious disease included poor living conditions, spoiled or improperly prepared foods, nonexistent surgical equipment, and surgeons not washing their hands before surgery. African American troops died from disease at a higher rate than European American troops.[35] This was the result of even poorer living conditions, unhealthy posts such as being quartered in wetlands or swamps, an unhealthy diet, substandard supplies and rations, the indifference of Union command, and fewer doctors being available to treat Black soldiers. Herbert Aptheker, a prominent historian of African American history, tabulated the death figures by combat and disease for four units of the US Colored Troops (the 29th Connecticut, 5th Cavalry, 54th Massachusetts, and 55th Massachusetts) and found that 29 percent died in combat and 71 percent died from infectious disease.[36] It is possible that this disparity resulted from the fact that Negro regiments did not enter combat until later in the war. However, the units included in Aptheker's paper saw their fair share of combat and suffered higher disease mortality than the average for all units.

In the winter of 1865, shortly after the war ended, a major smallpox epidemic emerged in Washington, DC, and spread across the nation. Newly freed people were disproportionately affected by the outbreak because they had virtually no housing and little food and were exposed to the elements. Smallpox is caused by the *Varicella* virus, which is airborne. Crowded conditions favor the spread of both airborne and waterborne pathogens. The smallpox epidemic spread through the upper South in 1863 and 1864, the lower South and the Mississippi Valley in 1865, and the Western territories, thus affecting Native Americans, between 1866 and 1868.[37] The spread of smallpox and other infectious diseases among the freed people was taken as evidence of their innate biological inferiority and further evidence that they would never be able to integrate into white society or govern themselves.

This worldview was held by many of the whites who worked in the Freedmen's Bureau. This was the US government agency tasked with helping the newly freed slaves and poor whites after the Civil War. A prominent member of the bureau was the polygenist Louis Agassiz. Polygeny, the notion that God created separate species of human beings and that only "Caucasians" were the descendants of Adam and Eve, was the prominent scientific theory of human diversity in the first part of the nineteenth century.[38] The Swiss-born naturalist originally had no contact with or thoughts about people of African descent until he arrived in the Americas in the 1850s. However, as part of his career plan, he purposefully injected himself into the "race" and slavery debate. Agassiz opposed slavery not because he felt it was morally wrong but because of his desire to rid the country of Africans. His theories of African inferiority deeply influenced his thinking and policy recommendations during his time at the Freedmen's Bureau.[39] The notion of the inherent inferiority of Africans was also supported by the growing popularity of social Darwinism (Herbert Spencer's idea that "survival of the fittest" determined one's lot in society) and the "Negro extinction" hypothesis of the latter half of the nineteenth century.[40]

The conditions faced by African Americans in the late 1800s and early 1900s were conducive to the spread of infectious disease. These factors included stress (which negatively influences cell-mediated immune responses), lack of adequate shelter and clothing, geographical proximity to disease vectors, poor nutrition, and poverty. Chief among these was poverty because it drove the other factors. Ongoing poverty resulted from the lack of desire on the part of European Americans to allow African Americans to improve their lot in the economy. Former slaveholders enacted a program to return African Americans to a state of peonage (e.g., sharecropping) in the "redeemed" South after Reconstruction ended. In the North, African Americans faced hostility from newly arriving European immigrants over dominance in the region's growing industries. In the West, African American migration was limited by the desire of European Americans to claim those lands for themselves.

Thus, the disparities in infectious disease experienced by African Americans should not have been surprising, nor should those disparities ever have been ascribed to the innate character of African Americans. This can be understood by examining two infectious diseases transmitted by quite different means. *Mycobacterium tuberculosis*, which causes tuberculosis, has been known since ancient times. The Greeks called the disease it causes *phthisis*, which means to "waste away." In the nineteenth century, it was widespread and called consumption. In 1850, Samuel Cartwright (the prominent southern physician who invented the disease "draptemania") declared that Black consumption was different from white consumption.[41] Transmission of *M. tuberculosis* is airborne and facilitated by droplets emitted during coughing. However, exposure to the bacterium does not necessarily result in infection. Only about 25 percent of those exposed will progress to primary infection, and only about 10 percent of those will develop active tuberculosis. Some nonairborne transmission also takes place but is much rarer than airborne transmission.[42] Tuberculosis is still a major problem worldwide, and it is estimated that one-third of the global population is infected. World Health Organization estimates show that the disease is most prevalent in the poorest nations, with 193 and 280 cases per 100,000 people per year reported in Africa and Asia, respectively.[43]

Modern research has demonstrated several risk factors associated with tuberculosis infection, including stress, nutritional status, occupation, tobacco smoking, poverty, and diabetes mellitus. Several of these easily explain the disparity observed by socially defined race in the 1800s. During the Jim Crow era in the American South, the mortality rate for African Americans was 450 per 100,000—three times the rate for European Americans.[44] At that time, the rates for syphilis (caused by *Treponema pallidum*, a sexually transmitted pathogen) were also much higher in African American communities. The medical narrative at the turn of the twentieth century located this problem in the "inferiority" of the Negro, either by creation or evolution. For example, a Detroit physician named W. T. English wrote, "The Negro is the lowest species in the Darwinian hierarchy." Others claimed the cause was the strong sexual appetite of the Negro and a complete lack of morality within the race. Dr. English warned of the danger of Negro men's perverted desire for white women.[45] It is hard to know how many white physicians held views like these, but these statements are entirely consistent with the racial ideology of the time.

In the early 1930s, the Rosenwald Fund, a philanthropic organization based in Chicago, became concerned with the prevalence of syphilis in the American Negro population. This interest was not entirely charitable in that, similar to concerns with tuberculosis, public health physicians understood that high rates of disease in Negroes posed a threat to whites. Through research, the US Public Health Service (USPHS) learned that socioeconomic factors played a major role in determining disease prevalence—as opposed to socially defined race. Dr. Taliaferro Clark, a consultant for the Rosenwald Fund, observed that the prevalence of syphilis seemed to be connected with poverty. The fund had studied syphilis prevalence in six rural counties: Albemarle, Virginia; Pitt, North Carolina; Bolivar County, Mississippi; Tipton County, Tennessee; Glynn County, Georgia; and Macon County, Alabama. Macon was the poorest of the counties. Macon's prevalence was 40 percent compared with just 10 percent and 13 percent in Albemarle and Pitt, respectively. The USPHS concluded that it was access to social, economic, and educational opportunities that was driving that difference.[46]

What most people think they know about the study of untreated syphilis in Macon County—the Tuskegee Study of Untreated Syphilis in the Negro Male—is derived from the book *Bad Blood* by the historian James H. Jones, originally published in 1981 (an updated and expanded edition was published in 1993).[47] The study was also dramatized in the 1997 HBO film *Miss Evers' Boys* starring Alfre Woodard and Laurence Fishburne. This study was conducted by the US Public Health Service (USPHS) from 1932 to 1972). It was designed to study the progression of untreated syphilis in the Negro male (even though studies of untreated syphilis already existed derived from Norwegian males). When the study began, treatment for syphilis was generally ineffective and used toxic compounds such as mercury. However, patients were never informed that they had an infectious disease, that it was transmitted sexually, and that treatment was available. Worse, after penicillin became available, they were still not offered treatment. The USPHS did offer the participants "burial insurance."[48]

The historian Allan Brandt summarized the ethical problems with this study:

(1) The medical profession adhered to the Negro extinction hypothesis, particularly the notion that the race would go extinct in the twentieth century as a result of vice, crime, and disease—particularly venereal disease.
(2) Physicians discounted the role of the social determinants of the disease.
(3) Physicians did not believe that better medical care would alter the fate of the Negro (i.e., extinction).
(4) The physicians who initiated and continued the study accepted the beliefs espoused by the Negro extinction hypothesis.
(5) In the 1950s, penicillin had become the accepted and preferred treatment for syphilis, but it was not given to the men in the study.[49]

Brandt further argued that the study was ethically compromised because the USPHS did not tell the men being studied that they were part of an experiment; the men were participating under the guise of being treated but were not actually being treated; the USPHS prevented the men from getting treatment; getting the men to the autopsy stage of the study required deceptions and inducements; and not treating the men left their entire community at risk of acquiring syphilis.[50]

However, it has been argued that the treatment of the role of the doctors involved in the Tuskegee study has not been balanced. Specifically, it has been claimed that the descriptions of the white and Black doctors in popular accounts unfairly attribute bias to the white physicians.[51] For example, the prominent African American biological anthropologist William Montague Cobb was not overly critical of the Tuskegee study. Cobb commented on the study shortly after its conclusion in 1972 and pointed out that when the study began in 1932, whether untreated patients survived longer than treated patients was a valid scientific question. This was so because the standard treatments at the time used mercury compounds. Mercury is toxic to both animals and bacteria. Patients who received mercury-based treatment had a mortality rate 10 to 20 percent higher than those not treated. Further, when penicillin was introduced to treat syphilis in the 1950s, its effects were uneven: some patients responded, whereas others did not. It was also clear that by 1973, rates of venereal disease were rising despite the use of penicillin. While Cobb did not yet know this, it was most likely because of the spread of antibiotic-resistant genes resulting from the overprescription of antibiotics. Finally, Cobb thought that there was no evidence that anyone had been subjected to unavoidable harm in the Tuskegee study.[52]

The many ethical shortcomings of the Tuskegee study played a major role in the development of principles for the responsible conduct of research by professional scientific societies.[53] The harm caused by the study and the reporting of its problems is still with us. Its impact can be seen in the ease with which African Americans can be seduced by pseudoscientific claims about biomedical research, such as that vaccines cause autism, vaccines are ineffective and manufactured only for profit, and the medical establishment is making organized attempts at genocide in the African American community. During the COVID-19 pandemic, I had to deal with these fallacies in my own family. Recognizing the problem, I made sure that pictures were taken of me receiving my first shot of the Moderna vaccine. I also worked with the Episcopal Diocese of North Carolina and made a video spot to urge people to get vaccinated.

HIV AND RACE

The first case of acquired immunodeficiency syndrome (AIDS) in the United States was confirmed in 1981. There, it was first recorded in men who have sex with men who developed rare forms of cancer and pneumonia. The virus responsible for the disease, human immunodeficiency virus (HIV), was identified shortly thereafter. Originally, this virus was almost always fatal (my brother died of the disease in 1997). Very few doctors recognized the magnitude of the pandemic that would result from HIV transmission.

Data from 1990 to 2008 show that the greatest number of HIV infections, about 23.5 million, occurred in sub-Saharan Africa. This amounted to about 5 percent of the population, of which most were women. This is in contrast to the rest of the world, where most infected people are men. The history of HIV transmission helps explain this difference. It has been established that around 1940, the oldest human immunodeficiency virus, HIV-2, jumped from primates to humans. However, some sources claim that the jump was made in the 1930s.[54]

The first documented case occurred in Kinshasa, Democratic Republic of the Congo, in 1959. There, a seemingly healthy man walked into a clinic to give blood for a Western-backed study of blood diseases. Twenty-five years later, in the 1980s, researchers studying the spread of AIDS took a second look at the blood.[55] They discovered that the sample contained HIV, the virus that causes AIDS.[56]

The rapid spread of HIV on the African continent can be linked to the apartheid labor system in South Africa that lasted from 1948 to 1990. Around the mining camps where many African men worked, isolated from their partners and families for months at a time, bars and brothels proliferated. The reliance of migrant miners on sex workers undoubtedly contributed to the spread of HIV across the continent.[57]

It is highly likely that sex workers played a significant role in the spread of HIV to the United States. It is important to recognize that sex work is not performed willing for profit. Indeed, it is a symptom of the worst forms of social injustice forced onto poor people, mainly women, LGBTQ+ individuals, and sometimes children. Sex workers are typically maintained in the trade by violence and coercion, and the profits go to the pimps and corrupt law enforcement officials who allow the trade to persist around the world. Molecular evolution–based evidence strongly suggests that HIV entered the United States via Haiti, whose first cases were identified in 1978 and 1979. This is just about the same time of the earliest reports of AIDS in the United States.[58] The original subtype of the HIV virus that emerged in Africa is designated as subtype D. The subtype that established the HIV pandemic in the Western Hemisphere is subtype B. Using archived samples from Haiti, researchers demonstrated that the so-called tree of relatedness (or phylogenetic tree) of all HIV sequences in the Western Hemisphere started with a branch separating subtypes D and B. The most ancient of the subtype B sequences are of Haitian origin and have likely existed on the island since the early 1960s. The secondary outbreaks from the Haitian strain occurred in Trinidad and Tobago, and a group identified as the "pandemic strains" occurred in the United States, Canada, Argentina, Colombia, Brazil, Ecuador, the Netherlands, France, the United Kingdom, Germany, Estonia, Gabon, South Africa, South Korea, Japan, Thailand, and Australia.[59] The tree also indicates that HIV-1 B had likely been circulating in the United States since 1966, fifteen years before HIV and AIDS were recognized as an epidemic disease. The secondary outbreaks are consistent with the hypothesis that Haiti's "sex tourism" industry played a prominent role in the global outbreak.[60]

The transmission of HIV is best understood by the mechanism of infection. The infection begins when bodily fluid carries the virus from an infected person directly onto a mucous membrane or into the bloodstream of an uninfected person. HIV travels via semen, vaginal and rectal secretions, blood, and breast milk. It can be transmitted via heterosexual and gay sex, oral sex, needle sharing, transfusion with contaminated blood, unsafe medical procedures, childbirth, and breastfeeding. HIV also replicates in the white blood cells (T cells) responsible for protecting the body from infection. The disease it causes, AIDS, does not develop until the body's T cell count is very low. Sexual transmission is facilitated by the fact that after an initial bought of flu-like symptoms, it takes time for the virus to deplete the body's T cell population, sometimes several years. This means that infected people may not know that they are carrying an infectious virus. Thus, when HIV began circulating in the United States, it was predominantly among men who have sex with men, many of whom did not know they were sick for quite a while. For example, in 1981, the estimated number of male infections was 18,600 compared to only 1,500 female infections.[61] This pattern held throughout the pandemic, with the following rates reported in 2012 among men who have sex with men: in London, 12 percent; in New York City, 18 percent; and in San Francisco, 24 percent. Among intravenous drug users, 2012 rates were as follows: in France, 12 percent; in Canada, 13 percent, and in the United States, 16 percent.

However, estimates of HIV infection also show that prevalence of infection differs by socially defined race. In 1981, 1985, and 2019, the numbers of HIV infections in the United States for Black people were 5,800, 38,800, and 14,300, respectively, compared to 11,100, 72,100, and 8,600 for white people in the same years.[62] To understand the disparity in infection rates, the rates must first be normalized by difference in population size. Doing so, the number of cases for white people in a population the same size as that of Black people yields 1,564, 10,112, and 1,686, respectively, in 1981, 1985, and 2019. Thus, the rates of infection in Black people in those years were 3.7, 3.8, and 8.5 times those of White people.

The 2019 numbers are particularly appalling when one considers that double- and triple-drug HIV therapy known as highly active antiretroviral therapy (HAART) was invented in 1996. HAART uses a combination of drugs including co-reception inhibitors, fusion inhibitors, reverse transcriptase inhibitors, integrase inhibitors, and protease inhibitors to slow the rate at which HIV can find mutations that confer resistance. The mutation rate of HIV is one of the highest ever recorded for any virus at about one per thousand base pairs per generation (1×10^{-3}). This is why—despite projections by US Secretary of Health and Human Services Margaret Heckler in 1984 that an HIV vaccine would be available within two years—no vaccine has ever been developed. However, if you challenge the virus to overcome three drugs, the probability of finding three such mutations is now 10^{-9} (the probability of each independent event multiplied). Early data suggested that among men with access to HAART, there was no difference in AIDS-related illness or death compared to men without access.[63] The problem seemed to be a combination of factors that led access to HAART to be determined by socially defined race, especially for women.[64] Black and Brown people, particularly women, did not receive equitable access to high-quality care for HIV because they suffered disproportionately from poverty and low health literacy.

From all the cases of infectious disease discussed here, we can see that the differential rates of sickness and death suffered by African Americans since the nineteenth century have not been driven by any genetic deficiencies in this socially defined group. Rather, it is because of the structural racism in the United States, which has placed African Americans under conditions that guarantee worse outcomes compared to European Americans. I have been writing about this problem since the late 1990s, and I am hardly the first scholar to recognize the issue. W. E. B. Du Bois discussed it at the turn of the twentieth century in his description of the physical health of the Negro.[65] In the mid-twentieth century, William Montague Cobb worked to raise consciousness about the poor medical care that Black people received that contributed to early death.[66] At the turn of the twenty-first century, the Institute of Medicine (now known as the National Academy of Medicine) published a report addressing ongoing racial disparities in health care.[67] Indeed, the concept is well understood. So much so that a recent search I conducted in the National Library of Medicine database using the terms "social determinants of health" and "race" returned more than four thousand results. Thus, when the scholarly literature has conclusively demonstrated that the social determinants of health exist and that many determinants are negatively affected by structural racism, we are left with the paradox of why so many practicing physicians still believe—and teach—that the causes of the health disparities experienced by African Americans reside within their genetics.[68]

Chapter Six

BAD BLOOD

The Racialization of Sickle Cell Anemia

A Chicago cardiologist named James Harrick (1861–1954) made the first formal report of sickle cell anemia on November 15, 1910. His patient was a twenty-year-old dental student from Grenada named Walter Clement Noel (1884–1916).[1] Noel had developed a condition later named "acute chest syndrome" for which he was treated at the Presbyterian Hospital in Chicago, where he was seen by Dr. Harrick and an intern named Ernest Irons. A blood test known as a blood smear showed that Noel had aberrant-shaped red blood cells. About three months later, a second case was described, this of a twenty-five-year-old woman treated at the University of Virginia.[2] Her blood smear was also indicative of sickle cell, but the physicians thought she was suffering from a peculiar case of pernicious anemia. The third case came from a female patient with a blood smear that also showed elongated and sickle-shaped blood cells.[3] The fourth case was investigated at the John Hopkins Hospital, and it was here that physicians realized that all previous cases had been in Negroes or Negroes with an admixture of "Caucasian" blood. This led to the supposition that the trait was inherited and limited to the Negro race. And it was here that the term *sickle cell anemia* (SCA) was first used.[4]

Consistent with the medical thinking of the time, SCA was viewed in the general context of presumed Negro inferiority. It was thought that "Negro blood" caused the disease.[5] Then, blood played the role of genes in today's science. Thus, as the disease was thought to be inherited, it was soon viewed as being a Mendelian dominant trait. It is important to note that at this point, there was no scientific reason to believe that SCA was caused by a dominant allele. Mendelian genetics was still a new science, and American geneticists were just beginning to deploy it as a research tool.[6] It was not yet widely taught as a subject in medical schools. The work of developing a volume of human genetics traits at the Eugenics Record Office had not begun in earnest, and the scientists there paid little to no attention to SCA.[7] There were no detailed pedigrees illustrating the transmission of the trait, which would have allowed physicians to determine whether the trait was dominant or recessive. Thus, the idea that SCA was caused by a dominant gene was due more to the inherent racial bias of white physicians, as well as their desire to protect the white race from Negro blood, than to rigorous scientific investigation.

Yet cases of SCA in white patients began to appear in 1925.[8] The historian Keith Wailoo has argued that these reports only substantiated the fear among white physicians that miscegenation might be spreading the supposedly dominant SCA gene into the white community. Wailoo provided the example of a doctor, M. A. Ogden, who proclaimed that "intermarriages between Negroes and white persons directly endanger the white race by transmission of the sickling trait." A few years later, another white physician argued even more vehemently of the danger: "Its occurrence depends entirely on the presence of Negro blood."[9]

That these ideas were driven by bigotry and not science is further evidenced by the fact that enough population genetic theory already existed to demonstrate that the idea of the sickle trait being dominant could not be correct. Godfrey Hardy and Wilhelm Weinberg's theorem showing the expected frequencies of genotypes under random mating, referred to as the Hardy–Weinberg equilibrium, was published in 1908.[10] By 1931, Ronald A. Fisher, John Burdon Sanderson Haldane, and Sewall Wright had provided the mathematics demonstrating how allele frequencies were changed by natural selection.[11] Most importantly, Fisher had explained the evolution of dominance in 1931, and his argument made it clear that a disease-causing variant such as the one that caused SCA was highly unlikely to evolve dominance.[12] Even if SCA were caused by a dominant allele, existing theory easily demonstrated that it could not invade the white population. In short, this could not happen because the survivorship and reproduction of people with SCA in North America is much less than that of people without the trait. Nor could SCA increase in frequency among African Americans in North

America—counter to the belief of the 1920s. A Detroit physician claimed that as a Mendelian dominant condition, SCA must increase in prevalence in the Negro population. He opined, "Will not 'sickle cell anemia' then become a common condition?"[13] The error here is that the dominant or recessive expression of an allele has nothing to do with its capacity to increase in a population. The frequency of an allele is determined by its evolutionary fitness, defined as the product of its impact on an individual's survival and reproduction. SCA was already known to reduce both characteristics of individuals in North America because of the absence of high malaria transmission. Thus, even a rudimentary understanding of population genetics demonstrated that the frequency of SCA must be decreasing in North America. Indeed, Graham Serjeant, one of the foremost scholars of SCA, argued in 1985 that the frequency of SCA had dropped dramatically in African Americans, from 0.200 to 0.080 in approximately three hundred years, because the SCA variant reduced their survival in North America.[14]

THE POSTWAR POPULATION AND THE MOLECULAR GENETICS OF SICKLE CELL ANEMIA

By 1949, J. V. Neel and E. A. Beet had correctly established the genetics of SCA.[15] The trait was recessive, not dominant. Thus, to display SCA, one had to have received one copy of the allele from each biological parent. It was also noticed that the variant was present at elevated frequencies in malarial zones. Work in Uganda in East Africa had shown that the variant provided resistance against falciparum malaria (caused by the single-celled protozoan parasite *Plasmodium falciparum*, a.k.a. "the killer"). With the trait being recessive, only one population genetic model could account for its high frequency in malarial zones: heterozygous advantage. In this model, people not carrying the variant would have reduced survivorship and reproduction because of some other factor (in this case, malaria); heterozygous individuals would have the highest survival and reproduction (because of resistance to malaria); and individuals homozygous for the allele would have reduced survival and reproduction because of SCA. This resulted in frequencies of SCA compatible with those measured in malarial zone populations in Southern Europe, the Middle East, tropical Africa, and India.[16]

Shortly after the population genetics of SCA were worked out, the molecular basis of the disease was established. The Nobel Prize winner Linus Pauling and his team determined that the sickle cell protein (Hb$_S$)

moved at a different rate from that of the nonsickling protein (Hb$_A$) under electrophoresis.[17] Pauling, who understood the population genetics of SCA transmission, took a eugenic approach to its prevention. He did not call for the sterilization of those carrying the trait but spoke harshly about those who did not take precautions regarding the genotype of those they might marry.[18] In 1977, the molecular basis of the common form of sickle cell anemia was worked out.

Because hemoglobin must carry oxygen under various conditions throughout the human life cycle, different hemoglobin molecules operate in the embryo, fetus, and adult. During early embryonic life, epsilon, zeta, and some alpha chains compose the molecule. During the fetal stage, alpha and gamma chains operate; during postnatal life, alpha, beta, and some delta chains operate. The hemoglobin of adults is a globular molecule composed of two polypeptide (alpha and beta) chains. These are intricately folded around each other, producing a pocket containing an iron molecule (heme). In the nonsickled hemoglobin beta-chain molecule, glutamic acid (an amino acid) is encoded by the triplet GAG in the messenger RNA. In SCA, a single missense mutation replaces an A with a U so that the triplet instead reads GUG, and the messenger RNA encodes a valine as the amino acid. Valine is an uncharged amino acid, and glutamic acid is a charged amino acid. These different charges cause a different folding of the beta chain, which affects the three-dimensional structure of the entire hemoglobin molecule. Hemoglobin C is caused by a mutation at the same codon position but at the first nucleotide so that GAG becomes AAG, replacing glutamic acid with lysine (also uncharged). Hemoglobin D-Punjab results from glutamine replacing glutamic acid (GAG becomes CAG). Other rarer mutations can also cause sickle cell anemia, including double base substitutions, insertions, and deletions of nucleotides.[19]

By the 1950s, it was recognized that in tropical malaria zones, few individuals homozygous for SCA were living long enough to reproduce.[20] As mentioned, the population genetic mechanism at work here was heterozygote advantage, which resulted in a balanced polymorphism. Balanced polymorphism in this case meant that both the nonsickled and sickled variant would persist in the population as long as heterozygotes displayed greater fitness. Balanced polymorphism can result from several causes, including frequency-dependent selection (fitness depending on the genotypic and phenotypic composition of the population), varying fitness by environment (fitness depending on the environment), and heterozygote advantage (whereas the homozygous form is harmful, the heterozygote form confers a survival advantage).[21]

We now recognize that heterozygote advantage produces several balanced polymorphisms associated with disease resulting from adaptation against malaria across the globe.[22] The Hb_S variant is found at elevated frequencies in malaria zones from West and Central Africa, Southern Spain, Southern Italy, Sicily, Greece, the Saudi Peninsula, and India. Hb_C is relegated to West Africa, and it is virtually absent in Southern Africa, Saharan Africa, and high-altitude environments in East Africa where malaria transmission is low or absent, or where a different antimalarial adaptation predominates, such as alpha or beta thalassemia.

ADDITIONAL ANTIMALARIAL ADAPTATIONS

Thalassemia results from a beta-chain imbalance caused by inadequate chain synthesis. This is usually caused by a deletion within either the alpha or beta gene. Thalassemia is classified by which chain is underproduced, alpha or beta. Alpha thalassemia is found at varying frequencies in African, Chinese, Mediterranean, South East Asian, and Northern European populations. Beta thalassemia is also generally caused by deletions, but at least one inversion (a segment of the gene being inserted in the wrong direction) has also been recorded. Its distribution mirrors that of alpha thalassemia. Individuals who are heterozygous for these mutations showed increased survivorship against malaria infection. This is due to reduced parasite invasion of cells, enhanced immune clearance of infected red blood cells, and reduced parasite survival and growth in the red blood cells.[23]

Ovalocytosis is another antimalarial adaptation.[24] Its geographic range is limited to Southeast Asia, Papua New Guinea, Indonesia, and the Philippines. Ovalocytosis is caused by a twenty-seven-base-pair deletion in the *SLC4A1* gene located at chromosomal position 17q21. The red blood cells in this condition are rigid and lack the expression of many red blood cell outer membrane proteins, which results in their resistance to malarial invasion. This change in red blood cell architecture affects the cells' ability to carry oxygen, resulting in many of the same symptoms observed in SCA.[25]

G6PD deficiency is an antimalarial adaptation found mainly in Africa, Asia, the Middle East, and Latin America.[26] It is currently estimated to affect about four hundred million people and is caused by more than two hundred mutations in the *G6PD* gene, located on the X chromosome (Xq28).[27] Most of the mutations are missense mutations that cause a reduction of the G6PD enzyme's ability to catalyze the first reaction in the pentose phosphate pathway. This is critical because this step is the only nicotinamide adenine dinucleotide phosphate (NADPH)-generating process in mature red blood cells. This is an essential co-enzyme for a variety of cellular process and without this molecule, red blood cells have no defense against oxidative damage. Of course, oxidative damage occurs in these cells because their very purpose is to carry oxygen to the body's tissues. This means that G6PD deficiency commonly results in drug-, food-, or infection-based hemolytic anemia or neonatal jaundice. Ingestion of fava beans is one of the most common causes of acute hemolytic anemia. The condition was discovered in 1956 as the result of an adverse reaction to the antimalarial drug primaquine.

Because the *G6PD* gene is found on the X chromosome, males are more likely to display the trait since they have only one X chromosome; females will display the trait only if they receive it from both biological parents. The frequency of *G6PD* mutations varies in malarial zones from 0.01 to as high as 0.20. Very high frequencies (closer to 0.20) occur in African, Middle Eastern, and Southeast Asian zones, while frequency in the Western Hemisphere is correlated with the past movement of enslaved people, which also brought mosquitoes and malaria parasites to the West.[28]

A HEALTH DISPARITY IN ANTIMALARIAL ADAPTATION

The common association of SCA with "Blackness" results from the simple fact that those who were enslaved to build America originated in the malarial zones of West and Central Africa. However, antimalarial adaptations exist wherever humans encounter malaria. Malarial transmission to humans began with the ancient development of agriculture, and as humans moved across the globe, they brought the malaria vectors, mosquitoes, and the various species of malaria (*Plasmodium* spp.) with them. However, significant migration to the United States from East Asia did not begin until the late nineteenth century and from the Middle East and India not until the twentieth century. These populations still represent a much smaller percentage of Americans than those of primarily recent African descent. Therefore, in their daily practice, physicians are still much more likely to come across people of African descent with SCA than East Asians with thalassemia or Middle Easterners or East Indians with SCA. Currently, about one hundred thousand Americans suffer from SCA, the vast majority of whom are of

African descent.[29] In the absence of determined education in medical or population genetics, it is easy even for nonracist physicians to commit the ascertainment fallacy of associating SCA with Blackness.

THE TERRIBLE SUFFERING CAUSED BY SICKLE CELL ANEMIA

As SCA results from deformed red blood cells that impair oxygen flow to the body's tissues, its clinical manifestations are horrible. It reduces and damages the function of the bone marrow, liver, spleen, gut, kidneys, eyes, gonads, bones, and joints, as well as the pulmonary, immune, cardiovascular, and nervous systems. It also negatively affects pregnancy and conception. One of its most severe symptoms is periodic crises of extreme pain known as vaso-occlusive episodes.[30] One of the most common causes of death associated with SCA is acute chest syndrome; this is what killed Clement Noel in 1916. The life expectancy of Americans with SCA increased over the twentieth century from an average of less than five years in 1910 to about forty-five years in 2000 (figure 6.1). This increase in life expectancy resulted mainly from the introduction of antibiotics to treat the recurrent infections associated with the disease. A dramatic increase in lifespan was observed after the Nixon administration passed the National Sickle Cell Anemia Control Act of 1972, which resulted in increased funding for research on treatment (although this was still inadequate for the need).[31] Other important treatment

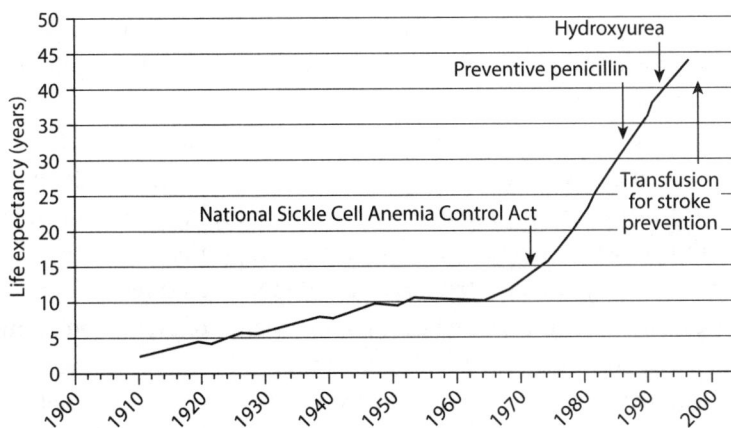

FIGURE 6.1. Increases in life expectancy in people with sickle cell anemia over the course of the twentieth century Source: K. Wailoo, "Sickle Cell Disease—A History of Progress and Peril," *New England Journal of Medicine* 376, no. 9 (2017): 805-807.

developments included the use of preventive penicillin and hydroxyurea (which makes red blood cells bigger and more flexible) in the 1980s, as well as the use of blood transfusions to prevent stroke in the 1990s.[32]

The extremely painful vaso-occlusive episodes (VOEs) that people with SCA experience result primarily from the blocking of capillaries by the sickled red blood cells. The pain results from ischemia (lack of oxygen) and inflammation. VOEs can last for hours or days, and 20 percent of people with SCA experience a VOE at least once a month. Of these, another 20 percent will develop acute chest syndrome within three days of being hospitalized.[33] Acute chest syndrome is treated with opioid and nonopioid analgesics.[34]

However, people with SCA continue to be harmed in many ways, including a lack of standardized care, misguided distrust of reported pain levels, inappropriate response times for people suffering from VOEs, and stigma toward people with SCA. These combine to result in significant undertreatment of pain.[35] This undertreatment is also influenced by a persistent false belief among physicians that Black people have greater pain tolerance because of their supposedly less sensitive nerves.[36] Many also falsely believe that people with SCA are drug seekers who misuse opioids. However, there is little evidence of this: only 0.5 percent of opioid overdose–related deaths from 1999 to 2013 occurred in people with SCA. The number of opioid-related deaths among people with other chronic pain conditions such as fibromyalgia (which are not experienced predominantly by people of African descent) are more than five times higher.[37] The stigmatization of people with SCA can also become self-imposed after experiencing it from relatives, the community, or health care providers. Stigma often appears in the form of microaggressions as when people with SCA are told that they are overreporting their pain or when they are accused of drug seeking.

Undoubtedly, the greatest harm inflicted on people with SCA results from the chronic underfunding of biomedical research into the development of better treatments and pain management. For example, in the United States cystic fibrosis, which is a rarer disease that disproportionately affects people of Northern European ancestry, has received more than three times as much funding from 2000 to 2018. In 2020, the prevalence of cystic fibrosis in the United States was thirty thousand individuals, while the prevalence of SCA was one hundred thousand.[38] Funding from the National Institutes of Health for cystic fibrosis research has always been greater than for SCA (in 2004, $128 million versus $90 million). In 2018, despite the three-fold-greater prevalence of SCA, the Trump administration reduced funding for SCA-related research to $76 million but left cystic fibrosis funding untouched.[39] Also, there are far fewer specialized treatment centers for SCA compared with those for rarer diseases such as hemophilia (which, again, is not suffered differentially by people of African descent). In the United States in 2023, there were 140 hemophilia treatment centers but just seventy-seven for SCA. The prevalence of hemophilia in the United States is only half that of SCA (about fifty thousand individuals).[40] Further, dedicated SCA treatment centers are scare in both rural and poor communities, which is significant when you consider the distribution of African American communities in the South and that the median income of African Americans is only one-tenth that of European Americans. Thus, many people with SCA have limited health insurance. It has been demonstrated that people receiving public aid, such as Medicaid, suffer worse outcomes than those with private insurance coverage.[41] The ineffectiveness of poor insurance for people with SCA results from the fact that this disease requires constant and expensive medical treatment.

DISTANT WATER FOR A NEARBY FIRE

The standard of care for SCA includes blood transfusions, bone marrow transplants, and drug therapy. However, blood transfusions and bone marrow transplants are limited in their efficacy, and the latter is limited by the availability of compatible donors. Up to 25 percent of people with SCA patients cannot find a suitable match for their bone marrow tissue. The US Food and Drug Administration has only approved four drugs for the treatment of the acute complications of SCA: hydroxyurea, L-glutamine, crizanlizumab, and voxelotor.[42] Hydroxyurea works by increasing the production of fetal hemoglobin, which in turn prevents the sickling of red blood cells. It has also been shown to reduce acute and chronic complications, hospitalization rates, and length of hospital stay, in addition to reducing the frequency of VOEs by up to 50 percent. It also reduces the risk of acute chest syndrome, stroke, and other complications. Yet, as with all medications, response to this drug varies considerably. Response is influenced by the patient's genetics, age, baseline hemoglobin levels, and comorbidities. L-glutamine is a naturally occurring amino acid that works against SCA by increasing the availability of glutathione. Glutathione protects red blood cells against oxidative damage and thereby prevents sickling. This medication has been shown to reduce VOEs by up to 25 percent and alleviate pain, thus improving the quality of life of people with SCA.[43] Crizanlizumab is an antibody against P-selectin, a transmembrane protein that plays a role in inflammation, causing white blood cells to adhere to platelets and the endothelium of blood vessels. In SCA, white blood cells adhering to these surfaces promotes the clogging of blood vessels, which is a main cause of the pain crises endured by people with SCA. Crizanlizumab has been shown to reduce VOEs by about 45 percent. Finally, voxelotor inhibits the polymerization of deoxy-sickle hemoglobin, resulting in an increase in the oxygen affinity of the hemoglobin. This improves blood flow and reduces sickling. This drug has been shown to decrease the incidence of VOEs by at least 65 percent.[44] Together, these four drugs have improved the quality of life of people with SCA, but none is a cure.

However, new technologies are being developed that are at least technically promising to cure single-gene disorders. In 2014, a new tool known as the "CRISPR-Cas9 nuclease system" was discovered (CRISPR: clustered regularly interspaced short palindromic repeats; Cas9: CRISPR-associated protein 9). This system evolved in bacteria as a means of protection against bacteriophages and self-replicating plasmids, and the enzymes involved can be directed to rewrite a nucleotide sequence. Jennifer Doudna and Emmanuelle Charpentier were awarded the Nobel Prize in Chemistry in 2020 for their recognition that this system can be deployed to engineer nucleotide sequences.[45]

Not long after the discovery of CRISPR-Cas9, it was proposed as a tool for curing single-gene disorders by simply rewriting a portion of the affected gene. This could be achieved in the germ line, as was demonstrated by the Chinese researcher He Jiankui in 2018. However, Jiankui's work was uniformly condemned by the international scientific community for reopening the gates of eugenics, and a moratorium has been recommended on human germ-line editing.[46] Of course, there is no way to enforce such a recommendation, so we really have no idea whether such work is being conducted in secret by researchers without an aversion to eugenics. This concern is of continued importance for SCA because in the United States, physicians are still attempting to force unwanted sterilizations on African American women with SCA.[47]

However, to address SCA, it is not necessary to conduct germ-line gene editing. Red blood cells are produced in the bone marrow by hematopoietic stem and progenitor cells (HSPCs). The CRISPR-Cas9 system has already been used to rewrite the genome of these cells. This was achieved via a variety of delivery systems, including physical methods (microinjection and electroporation), viral vectors (HTV1, LV, AdV, AAV), and nonviral vectors (cationic polymers, liposomes, lipid nanoparticles, cell-penetrating peptides, gold nanoparticles, exosomes). The system can be incorporated via plasmid (a small self-replicating circular piece of DNA that originated in bacteria), messenger RNA, or ribonucleoprotein complex.[48] All have benefits as well as potential harms. For example, the use of any viral vector raises the potential that the virus may re-evolve the capacity to self-replicate. In such a scenario, it is likely that the patient would be severely harmed or even die from the procedure. Research on the rewriting of DNA to cure SCA has focused on different genetic systems with the goal of either changing the sickled beta chain into a nonsickled chain by repairing the mutations or changing the DNA promoter sequence to produce fetal hemoglobin (gamma-globin) and stop producing beta-globin. This work has also been conducted on people with transfusion-dependent beta thalassemia.[49] Thus far, the techniques have worked as designed. In addition, there have been few instances of off-target gene editing, a problem that can occur any time a gene-editing system is deployed and that must be evaluated to determine the safety of the technique. For example, in work my colleagues have done using the pORTMAGE plasmid to engineer genetic changes in the bacterium *Escherichia coli*, we found major examples of off-site editing that had never been reported by others using this system.[50]

So far, data on improvement in clinical outcomes has been reported for about two hundred people with SCA who have received HSPCs edited by CRISPR-Cas9 methods.[51] These studies have shown that patients display high levels of gene editing, increases in fetal hemoglobin distributed across cells, engraftment (altered and transplanted cells operating as intended), transfusion independence, and a reduction in VOEs (and in at least one case, the elimination of VOEs). However, the methods have not completely eliminated the adverse events associated with SCA. Of course, given the multifaceted manifestation of the disease, this is not unexpected.

So far, CRISPR-Cas9 technology is showing great promise for alleviating and maybe at some point eliminating the symptoms of SCA and thalassemia. If you have not already figured it out, the issue going forward is not the technology itself but its cost. In February 2024, the American Academy of Family Physicians stated that the cost of this type of therapy would put it out of reach for most Americans. The list price for one course of Casgevy, the first CRISPR-Cas9-based therapy for transfusion-dependent beta thalassemia is about $2.2 million.[52] This is more than the expected lifetime cost of standard

SCA treatment of $1.7 million. In addition, because HSPCs have limited lifespans, more than one course of CRISPR-Cas9-based treatment would be required across a patient's life time. It is not clear that insurance companies would be willing to pay more than what they do for standard treatment. Further, as most people with SCA and thalassemia reside in the poorer nations of Africa, they will most likely never receive gene-targeted treatments.

To address the disparity in gene therapy for vulnerable populations, in 2024, the Biden–Harris administration has announced that sickle cell disease would be the first focus of the Cell and Gene Therapy Access Model. This program is meant to increase access to cell and gene therapies and lower health care costs for those who need the treatments the most. The program is led by the Centers for Medicare & Medicaid Services Innovation Center. It will test outcomes-based agreements for groundbreaking cell and gene therapies. If it works, the best outcomes-based agreements will increase affordable access to potentially lifesaving and life-changing treatments.[53] The administration planned for access to the program to begin in 2025 with the goal of expanding the program to other types of cell and gene therapies in the future. Of course, the elephant in the room is whether the Trump administration will continue the program—or, if it does continue, whether it will be continued equitably to address genetic diseases whose prevalence is higher in nonwhites. Given Trump's history, it is highly likely that in his new administration, SCA will not be given any priority and funding to advance treatment will disappear. Furthermore, given the general cuts to the federal workforce (~10,000 employees) associated with Health, and Human Services (HHS), we can expect that research and care for these diseases will be eroded.[54]

Chapter Seven

CANCER IS UNFAIR

Almost all of us know someone who has been ill or died from cancer. This is not a coincidence. Cancer is a part of who we are; we couldn't be here without it. So the question must be asked: if cancer is so much a part of who we are, why do some groups suffer from this disease more than others? My grandfather Lewis died of prostate cancer. My father, Joseph Sr., was treated for prostate cancer. And I am most likely carrying genetic variants that predispose me to prostate cancer. This is not because I am Black. It's because these variants are inherited in my family. Everyone reading this is carrying genetic variants that could result in their being diagnosed with cancer. If you live long enough, you will certainly develop cancer. However, developing it and dying from it are not the same thing. When a person dies and during autopsies, physicians typically record the primary cause of death.[1] And many people who die from heart disease or some other late-age cause of death also have various cancers in their bodies.

To understand why everyone is carrying genetic variants that predispose them to cancer, we have to understand what the disease is. Cancer is not just one disease but rather a suite of diseases characterized by uncontrolled cell division and the spread of cells in the various tissues of multicellular organisms. Neoplasms (benign cancers), such as skin moles, are localized and stay so. Colon polyps are an example of premalignant (precancerous) neoplasms. These do not destroy or invade other tissues but can evolve to do so. The most dreaded forms of cancer are the malignant neoplasms that produce cells that can disperse and then invade and colonize other tissues. These often kill the host organism.[2]

At its most basic level, cancer can be thought of as a rebellion of specific cell lineages against the host organism. And why shouldn't they rebel? What exactly do these cells achieve by staying part of a collective? While most people take the existence of multicellular organisms for granted, evolutionary biologists do not. It took three-quarters of the history of life on Earth for multicellularity to evolve. In October 2023, I participated in a podcast exploring this subject.[3] The other guests included my colleague, Jeffery Barrick, a specialist in experimental evolution; William Ratcliff, an evolutionary biologist; and Ben Stanger, a cancer researcher. It was a spirited discussion, and we all agreed that the fact that the evolution of multicellularity took so long to develop illustrates that there is no simple logic that forces single cells to give rise to multicellular organisms.[4] This is still one of the big unsolved questions in evolutionary biology, one that experimental evolution methods are just beginning to work out.[5]

A key innovation that arose from the evolution of multicellularity was the separation of the germ and somatic lines during development. Germ cells give rise to the ovaries and testes in animals that reproduce sexually. These in turn produce the gametes used to produce the next generation. The somatic line produces the cells that do the work that makes the organism's survival and reproduction possible. These include the tissues that make up the nerves, muscles, bones, digestive track, internal organs, and skin. These cells give up their ability to reproduce to produce the functioning body that makes the gametes that carry the genome of an individual organism into the next generation. The analogy that explains this best is that a chicken is just an egg's way of making another egg (discussed in chapters 1 and 2). This can evolve because a multicellular organism can produce many more copies of its genome per generation than a single-celled organism can by binary fission. The latter is constrained to producing just twice the copies of its genome per generation (a two-fold increase). On the other hand, a multicellular female fruit fly can lay thirty eggs a day and has an average lifespan of forty days. This amounts to a possible 1,200 offspring, of which half the genome originates in the female parent. So, in one generation, the copies of the fruit fly's genome can increase six-hundred-fold. The cost for this, however, is senescence (aging) (discussed in chapter 2).

CANCER IS A DISEASE OF MAINTENANCE

In chapter 1, I discussed different types of disease in an evolutionary context. Diseases of maintenance are those for which the cost of preventing disease are too great in the context of improving an individual's fitness (i.e., differential reproductive success). The age-specific nature of cancer prevalence and mortality illustrate this well. Figure 7.1 shows the prevalence of all cancers in Canadians by biological sex in 2018.[6] The prevalence of cancer in this population clearly increases with age, and this is true across the globe. Figure 7.2 shows the mortality rate for all cancers in Americans in 2018. The inflection point at which mortality rates begin to climb away from zero (between ages one and thirty-four years) is at age forty years. This is significant because the average age of menopause onset in the United States is estimated to be around fifty years.[7] Male reproductive senescence closely follows that of females, and even if their reproductive competence (their ability to manufacture sperm) lasts longer, males of advanced age rarely sire offspring. Humans are unique among animals for having such a long postreproductive life span (see chapter 2). For example, in fruit flies, the day a female fly lays her last egg is usually the day she dies.[8] There is no significant difference between male and female lifespan in laboratory-reared flies.

Natural selection generally favors adaptations that improve reproduction, often at the cost of maintenance. Thus, mutations that negatively affect survivorship and reproduction during the developmental and reproductive

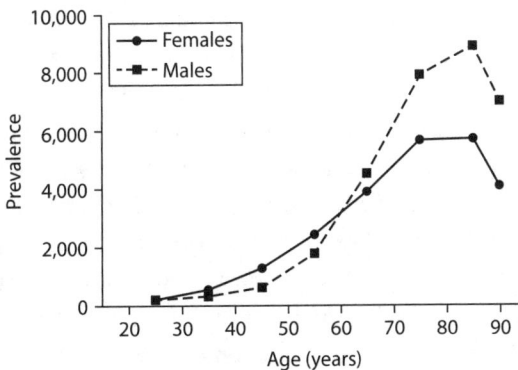

FIGURE 7.1. Cancer prevalence by age in Canada, 2018 *Source*: C. Yao and J. M. Billete, "Short-Term Cancer Prevalence in Canada, 2018," *Health Reports* 33, no. 3 (2022): 15–21.

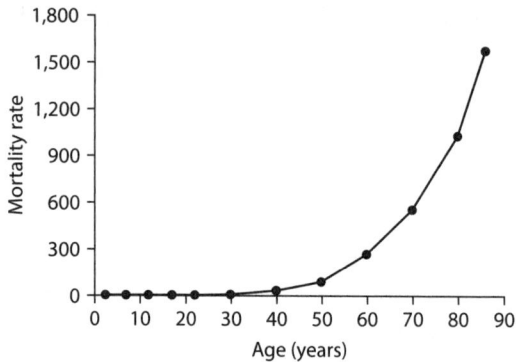

FIGURE 7.2. Age-specific cancer mortality in the United States, 2018 *Source*: M. Heron, "Deaths: Leading Causes for 2018," *National Vital Statistics Reports* 70, no. 4 (2021).

periods of an organism's life face strong negative natural selection (as discussed in chapter 2). Thus, germ-line mutations that cause cancer at early ages are very rare in humans. Such genes impair their own replication into the next generation; therefore, we would expect them to exist only at the rate of mutation (about 10^{-8}, or one per one hundred million per genome per generation in humans).[9] There is variation around this average rate. For example, a study of seven childhood cancers (acute lymphocytic anemia, acute myeloid leukemia, Burkitt-type lymphoma, chronic myeloid leukemia, Hodgkin's lymphoma, non-Burkitt-type lymphoma, and non-Hodgkin's lymphoma) over five years in Tehran, Iran, found only 328 cases in children under the age of fourteen years. Assuming equal rarity across conditions, the frequency of these cancers is 2.1×10^{-5}. Their rarity is predicted by the action of selection and the mutation rate, called the mutation–selection balance.[10]

On the other hand, natural selection has no power to eliminate deleterious alleles whose action occurs after an individual's net future expected reproduction has reached zero (see chapter 2). This realization developed over years of theoretical and experimental work on aging.[11] This is why the exponential increase in mortality rate for various diseases, including cancer, in humans is associated with the cessation of reproductive potential (e.g., menopause in women). The accumulation of such variants in our genomes can occur by two mechanisms: mutation accumulation and antagonistic pleiotropy (see chapter 2). If a variant has no impact on reproductive success in early life, its frequency will be governed by genetic drift (i.e., randomness).

However, any allele with a positive impact on early-life reproductive success will increase in frequency (until all of a population has it) despite any deleterious effect they might have in late life. This is the mechanism driving the ubiquity of cancer-capable genetic variants in the human genome. Cancers originate most frequently from the stem cells of tissues that require constant repair such as bone marrow, lung epithelia, the gut, and skin. The ability to repair tissue during development and reproduction is highly favored by natural selection (i.e., there is a positive effect in early life) even though it makes us vulnerable to uncontrolled cell growth and invasion after our reproductive lives have ceased (i.e., there is a negative effect in late life). This reasoning is supported by that fact that the most common cancers in American women are breast (32 percent), lung and bronchial (12 percent), colon and rectal (7 percent), and uterine (7 percent), whereas in American men, the most common are prostate (29), lung and bronchial (11 percent), colon and rectal (8 percent), and bladder (6 percent).[12]

During the developmental and reproductive periods of our lifespan, the mechanisms that keep rogue somatic cells from initiating tumors work really well. We have tumor-suppressor genes that control differentiation and eliminate damaged cells. If a cell begins to divide when it should not, it receives a chemical signal that makes it kill itself in a process known as apoptosis. If DNA is damaged inside a cell, a series of proteins can repair that damage. Both mechanisms are regulated by the p53 gene family (*TP53*, *TP63*, and *TP73*). The p53 protein is a transcription factor that is divided into five domains. Amino acids 1 to 55 contain two transactivation (increasing or stimulating gene expression) sequences. This is followed by a proline-rich domain involved in protein-to-protein interactions. Next is a DNA-binding domain, which is followed by a tetramerization domain (facilitates the formation of a molecule with four subunits), and finally a regulatory domain in which amino acid modifications such as methylation and acetylation regulate the protein's activity.[13] However, in later life, mutations in the p53 protein diminish its ability to carry out these processes. Immune surveillance of cancer cells is also at its highest during our development and reproduction phases. The immune system generally does not attack the body's own tissues; rather, it recognizes pathological cells with inappropriate metabolism, growth, and movement. Before our reproductive phase ends, the immune system eliminates or controls most tumor lineages so that they cannot progress to cancers. Again, mutations that weaken our immune surveillance mechanisms are not eliminated by natural selection if they occur after the reproduction phase of life ends.

In addition, the novel environments that we inhabit have increased the number of environmental factors that can cause mutations in somatic cells, such as air and water pollution, ultraviolet light, nuclear radiation, tobacco smoke, free radicals released from inflammatory processes, and novel substances such as per- and polyfluorinated alkyl compounds known as "forever chemicals." Such compounds are found in the blood of most Americans and are associated with certain cancers such as renal cell carcinoma.[14]

Exposure to carcinogenic compounds either by occupation or by residence is determined by socially defined race in the United States. This is discussed in detail in a 2007 report titled *Toxic Wastes and Race at Twenty*.[15] This report documents a historical location of toxic waste sites in poor communities by socially defined race. In addition, Black and Brown communities are exposed to greater amounts of PM2.5 particulate matter, associated with an increased risk of lung cancer, in air pollution.[16] The location of toxic waste sites in poor areas and the differential exposure to water and air pollution experienced by racialized communities may explain the relationship between residential segregation and racial disparities in cancer prevalence. It has been shown that among African Americans, living in segregated areas is associated with a higher likelihood of later-stage diagnoses, higher mortality rates, and lower survival rates for breast and lung cancers.[17] In addition to toxic physical environments, the cumulative stress of structural racism can also contribute to the biologic basis of differential gene expression at later ages (as will be discussed in chapter 8). Thus, while we all have a genetic predisposition to cancer at late age, some of us are more likely to be made sick and die from cancer owing to environmental circumstances.

GLOBAL CANCER INCIDENCE

The genetic elements that predispose us to cancer entered our genome long before the human species existed. For example, the simple unicellular eukaryotic group choanoflagellates that is the most likely precursor to animals has a p53 orthologue (a gene that first evolved in a common ancestor but evolved differently in its descendants). This is not found in bacteria, fungi, or plants.[18] The ancestor of humans and choanoflagellates probably existed about six hundred million to eight hundred million years ago. This means that when our species first evolved in Africa about three hundred thousand years ago, the genetic mechanisms regulating cancer already existed. Why, then, should any biological population or socially defined racial group differ in their predisposition to cancer? If such differences exist, do they relate to cancer in general or to specific cancers? Are differences in the prevalence of specific cancers driven by difference in genetics or differences in environmental exposure? The answer is that both genetic and environmental differences play a role in the pattern of cancer incidence we see in American society—but not in the simplistic racialized ways that most people, including many physicians, think.

Theory suggests that cancer variants driven by antagonistic pleiotropy should be fixed in all human populations. For example, the frequency of a risk variant in the *FGFR2* gene, which encodes the fibroblast growth factor receptor 2 protein, is pretty uniform around the globe. This variant is associated with a higher risk of postmenopausal breast cancer, but it is also associated with angiogenic (formation of new blood vessel) growth in the uterus in early life.[19] This relationship fits the definition of antagonistic pleiotropy. Using data from the dbSNP database (which includes data for Europeans, Africans, African Americans, Asians, East Asians, South Asians, and others), I computed the population subdivision statistic (F_{ST}) for this variant as 0.00075. F_{ST} measures how similar the frequency of alleles for specific genes are in subpopulations in a species. An F_{ST} this low means that pretty much every sample in the analysis has about the same frequency of the risk variant.

However, a significant polymorphism in some cancer-associated loci appears to exist. For example, the *TP53-R72P* variant has been well studied. This nomenclature means that at the seventy-second position of the TP53 protein, some populations have a proline (P) amino acid (more frequent in sub-Saharan Africans, with an average frequency of 0.685), and others have an arginine (R) amino acid (more frequent in Europeans, with an average frequency of 0.736). The R variant has been linked to more aggressive apoptosis, and the P variant has been linked to reduced fertility.[20] More aggressive apoptosis should be protective against the formation of cancer in early life, but there is no guarantee that this variant continues that protective role in late life. Indeed, one study of the role of the *TP53-R72P* variant in the survival of people with breast cancer found no such effect compared with those who did not carry the variant.[21] The role of the *TP53* gene in cancer prevention is complex. It harbors polymorphisms in at least 376 sites that appear to play different roles in allowing cancer formation in somatic cells.

Even more polymorphism in cancer-related variants should result from mutation accumulation. As these variants have no impact on reproductive success in early life, their frequency is determined by random chance. Thus, we would expect that the impact of these variants on cancer predisposition would vary by population as opposed to socially defined race. Thus, while both Swedes and Finns could be considered white, each population might have dramatically different frequencies in such variants by random chance, and the contribution of those variants to any cancer phenotype would also result in random patterns by socially defined race. For example, in 2019, breast cancer incidence in Sweden was 217.5 per 100,000 but only 58.9 in Crete; in 2013 in Russia, it was 47, and in 1999 in Finland, it was 76.[22] The fact that these estimates are from different years doesn't mean we can't compare them because the difference is too small to have caused significant changes in allele frequency. Human generation times are about thirty years, meaning that allele frequencies calculated in 1999 would be relatively the same in 2019.

However, the most important mutational process determining the onset of cancer occurs in somatic tissues. The accumulation of mutations in those tissues begins in development, continues through reproduction, and accelerates during senescence. There is a direct relationship between the number of divisions within a particular tissue and the accumulation of mutations in the cells that compose it.[23] Thus, cell types that undergo little cell division are less likely to produce tumors compared with cells derived from stem cells in tissues that are always undergoing division to replace damaged cells. Data shows that the mutational profile of normal cells differs within given individuals. Even normal cells have mutations that can cause the cell to lose replication control under certain circumstances; these are called driver mutations. Driver mutations most often appear in the following genes: *BRAF* (serine/threonine-protein kinase B-raf, which plays a role in communicating cell division signals from the cell membrane to the nucleus), *GNAS* (guanine nucleotide-binding protein G(s) subunit alpha isoforms XLas, which are involved in signaling pathways controlled by G-protein-coupled receptors), *PTPN11* (GRB2-associated binding protein 2, which acts with several membrane receptors to regulate multiple signaling pathways), *FOXA1* (hepatocyte nuclear factor 3-alpha, which acts in embryonic development to establish tissue-specific gene expression and the regulation of gene expression in differentiated tissues), *KRAS* (GTPase KRas, in which Ras proteins bind GDP with GTP and possess intrinsic GTPase activity), and *TP53*.

Environmental exposures play an important role in stimulating cell driver mutations to bring about cancer. A study in Finland showed that occupational exposure to mutagenic factors increased the risk of postmenopausal breast cancer. Risk was most accelerated by medium to high levels of ionizing radiation, human-made asbestos and vitreous fibers, aromatic hydrocarbon solvents, animal dust, gasoline, and diesel fuel exhaust.[24] A global examination of cancer incidence demonstrated that there is no consistent "racial" classification of cancer. In 2013, the age-adjusted incidence for tracheal, bronchus, and lung cancers for both sexes was lowest in sub-Saharan Africa (6.33), followed by East Africa (8.01), Central sub-Saharan Africa (12.77), North America (61.5), East Asia (64.68), and Central Europe (66.10). For breast cancer, age-adjusted incidence was lowest in Western sub-Saharan Africa (28.24), followed by East Asia (33.52), Eastern sub-Saharan Africa (33.67), Australia (European population, 91.12), North America (111.01), and Oceania (133.38). Other cancers such as colon and rectal, prostate, stomach, liver, cervical, non-Hodgkin lymphoma, esophageal, and leukemia show no consistent ranking by geography.[25] This data demonstrates that there is no geographically based genetic basis to cancer incidence. The ranking of cancers was not consistent by population or geographic region. The study from which this data was extracted proposed economic development as the main factor influencing incidence and type of cancer. It also demonstrated that a higher incidence of cancer is more the result of wealth and affluence than population genetics. In this regard, it is likely that people living in less developed regions of the world receive less exposure to environmental factors such as toxic chemicals, ionizing radiation, and inflammatory diets that generate driver mutations in somatic cells. An alternative explanation for the lower rates of cancer incidence in these nations is that other sources of death are obscuring cancer incidence rates or that in the poorest nations, cancer incidence is under-recorded owing to a lack of access to health care leading to people dying earlier in life, before cancers form.

CANCER DISPARITIES IN THE UNITED STATES

Cancer incidence and mortality data for the United States also shows no consistent pattern in socially defined race or ethnicity. Figure 7.3 shows the mean and standard error for age-specific cancer mortality for non-Hispanic Black and white individuals in the United States from 2015 to 2021 (all types of cancer were included). The data shows that the age-specific mortality of Blacks is statistically significantly higher than that of whites over that time period. An individual's likelihood of developing and dying from cancer is influenced by their genetics, their environment, and chance. As discussed, the genetics

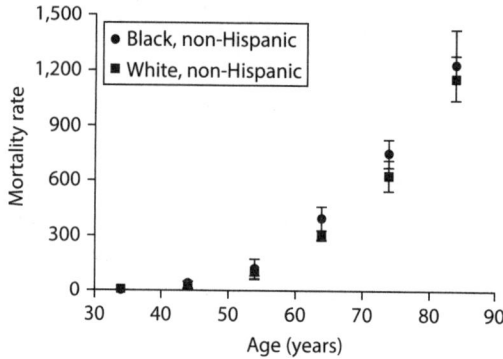

FIGURE 7.3. Cancer death rates for non-Hispanic Blacks and whites in the United States, 2015–2021

of the myriad of diseases that we call "cancer" is complex. Thus, the cancer phenotype is best understood via the tools of quantitative genetics.

Unfortunately, the notion of genetic differences between Black and white populations has dominated too much of the narrative concerning health disparities in cancer incidence and mortality. This notion is a fallacy. To understand why, we must review what we know about human population genetics. Any two people chosen at random from anywhere in the world will share anywhere from 99.4 to 99.9 percent of their genome in common. Any two people chosen at random from the continent of Africa will likely be more different from each other than two people chosen at random, one from Africa and one from Europe. This is because there is simply more genetic variation in Africa than in the rest of the world. African Americans (whom I define as the descendants of enslaved people in the United States) have, on average, 16 percent European ancestry, and in some states, such as Kansas, Washington, and West Virginia, European ancestry exceeds 25 percent on average.[26] So, while geographically based genetic variation exists in the human species, it does not coincide directly with the socially defined racial groups created by the legacy of colonialism, genocide, and slavery in the Western Hemisphere. Further, the existence of genetic differences is not a guarantee that any differences in a given trait are the result of genetic differences because environmental influences play a significant role in the production of phenotypes. Indeed, environmental influences play a major role in patterns of gene expression. A recent study examined whole-genome gene expression (transcriptome, which refers to the genes that are transcribed) in a diverse sample (731 people across five continents). The authors found that 92 percent of the variation of gene expression and 95 percent of the variation in gene splicing (which also influences gene expression) occurred within the populations.[27] This means that there was more variation in people from the same continent than between groups from different continents. This is important to understand because people often conflate continental origin with biological race. This is also important to understand in the context of cancer because the somatic mutations that drive cancer formation often result from the cumulative impact of environmental stressors altering patterns of gene expression. This is well illustrated in the case of breast cancer in the United States.

Melanoma of the skin is the most commonly diagnosed cancer in women in the United States, followed by breast cancer. It is also the second most common cause of cancer death (after lung cancer). It is the leading cause of death of African American and Hispanic women.[28] One recent study suggested that 30 percent of breast cancer cases result from potentially modifiable causes such as excess body weight, cigarette smoking, infectious disease (*Heliobacter pylori*, i.e., human herpes virus type 8), physical inactivity, and alcohol intake.[29] These "modifiable causes" are part of an individual's environment, but it is important to understand that there is often little a person can do to alter those factors, particularly those who are socially subordinated. Other ways to reduce the risk of death from breast cancer include improved mammography screening and advances in treatment. But, as you may expect by now, access to these interventions is strongly stratified by socially defined race and class in the United States.

One of the greatest contradictions in the breast cancer story is that while African American women have a lower incidence of breast cancer, they experience a higher death rate.[30] Incidence rates are higher in white women than in Black women (133.7 and 127.8 per 100,000, respectively, in 2022), but death rates are higher in Black women than in white women (27.6 and 19.7 per 100,000, respectively, in 2022). It has been argued that this disparity can be explained in part by the differential prevalence of subtypes of breast cancer in the two groups. Breast cancer subtypes are differentiated by the hormone receptors displayed on cell surfaces, particularly those for estrogen and progesterone (HR) and human epidermal growth factor (HER2). These receptors are critical because they allows genes within a cell to "understand" whether the host is actively reproductive or not. In 1993, I published a paper explaining the significance of reproductive signaling and the age-specific expression of deleterious genetic variants in mammals.[31] In short, the population genetic mechanisms that account for the evolution of aging—mutation accumulation and antagonistic pleiotropy—can work only if the negative genetic variants have a means of determining what life stage an organism is experiencing. A reduction in reproductive hormonal levels is the signal required to stimulate the expression of genetic variants that drive the transformation of somatic cells into tumor cells. Thus, cells not receiving signals from estrogen, progesterone, or human epidermal growth factor "perceive" that the host organism is past the reproductive phase of their life. In turn, the genetic cooperation of "selfish" elements that occurs during the developmental and reproductive stages of an organism's life ceases in the postreproductive stage, resulting in cancers and other dys-regulations of cell function.

The most aggressive form of breast cancer is called triple-negative (HR-negative/HER2-negative). In the United States, this is most common among Black women, occurring in 19 percent of Black women versus just 9 percent in white women. It is convenient to think that this difference in prevalence must result from genetic differences between Black and white women. How-ever, this explanation doesn't hold up when one considers that the rate of triple-negative breast cancer is 47 percent lower in women born in East Afri-can countries compared with US-born Black women.[32] The argument fails because it treats all women of African descent as if they are derived from a single population group. Women from West African countries living in the United States show rates of triple-negative breast cancer similar to those of African Americans. This makes sense because the African ancestry of Afri-can Americans is derived from West and Central Africa, not East Africa.[33] Remember, too, that African Americans also have European ancestry, which women recently immigrated from East and West Africa do not. In that regard, it is important to recognize that there are more clinically deleterious genetic variants in European Americans than in African Americans.[34]

However, evidence also shows that there is an important social envi-ronmental component associated with the likelihood of developing triple-negative breast cancer. In one study of 81,499 women, it was notable how many aspects of the social environments of women of European and Afri-can descent differed. For example, marital status was statistically signifi-cantly different between groups, with a much greater proportion of Black women being single and never married (31.9 percent > 13.7 percent) and a much greater proportion of white women being married (55.7 percent >

33.8 percent). A statistically significant difference in marriage rates was also found in women who were HR-positive (ER-positive and/or PR-positive) and HER-negative but not in those who were triple-negative (ER-negative, PR-negative, HER2-negative). This study found that Black women living in neighborhoods with a higher proportion of Black residents had a statistically lower probability of being diagnosed with triple-negative breast cancer than Black women living in neighborhoods with a lower proportion of Black residents. However, the relationship between neighborhood composition and socially defined race had no impact on white women. The study also found that neighborhoods with high socioeconomic status were protective against triple-negative breast cancer for both Black and white women.[35]

The single greatest indication that environmental—not genetic—factors drive mortality rate differences in breast cancer between Black and white women is most likely that before 1980, rates between the groups were similar and did not begin to diverge until the widespread dissemination of advances in early detection and treatment. The racial disparity peaked with a 40 percent difference in 2011.[36] This implies that the difference results from differences in breast cancer care: lower- versus higher-quality screening and treatment. The disparity in mortality rate was also found to be associated with the introduction of adjuvant endocrine therapy in the early 1980s. This therapy differentially benefited people with HR-positive breast cancer. Yet even here, HR-positive Black women had a 19 percent higher mortality rate despite a 22 percent lower incidence of this subtype of breast cancer.[37] It has also been shown that breast cancer mortality rates are associated with historical redlining and bias in home loan lending.[38] Last, a highly statistically significant difference exists in breast cancer mortality rate by state—in ways you likely would not imagine. Using cancer mortality rates grouped by former Confederate and Union states from 2016 to 2021, I found that the mortality rate was four times higher for Black women living in former Union states compared with Confederate states; this finding was statistically significant ($p = 0.004$). This difference cannot be explained by genetic differences between the Black population in those states.

Cancer is unfair. Disparities exist in both incidence and mortality by socially defined race. The genes that predispose us to cancer exist in all of us. Some play an indispensable role in our development, maintenance, and reproduction. Variants in genes whose action is beneficial in early life are favored by natural selection despite their deleterious effects later in life and are at high frequency in all world populations. Variants that cause cancer in early life are driven to very low frequencies by natural selection. Their frequency may also differ by population and thus may differ by socially defined race. However, cancer incidence and mortality are complex phenotypes strongly influenced by environmental forces. In modern industrialized societies, the number of environmental factors that can contribute to cancers (referred to as mutagens) is large. Differential exposure can result in differential cancer incidence. For example, malignant melanomas are more likely to occur in fair-skinned individuals, including those with ancestry from temperate and Arctic zones such as North Africans, Middle Easterners, Central and Northeastern Asians, and Indigenous North Americans. Because of admixture, African Americans can also display fair-skin phenotypes. Excess exposure to ultraviolet light, air pollution, and tobacco smoking can all drive mutations that cause lung cancer. Novel diets, including things such as cured meats and preservative, drive elevated rates of colon and rectal cancer. However, all these factors have social environmental components associated with structural racism in the United States that relate to cancer incidence and mortality. To make cancer more "fair," we must address these racialized inequalities.

Chapter Eight

RACE AND EPIGENOMICS

Nobody Knows the Trouble We've Seen

Nobody knows the trouble I've seen
Nobody knows but Jesus
Nobody knows the trouble I've seen
Glory, Hallelujah

LYRICS FROM THE NEGRO SPIRITUAL,
"NOBODY KNOWS THE TROUBLE I'VE SEEN"

Social subordination is real, and it is part of the biology of nearly all social species. Its impacts on the survival and reproduction of individuals within a species have been well documented in the field of biology. Social status in both early life and adulthood alters an organism's physiology, disease risk, and lifespan.[1] This is true in humans, and the experience of African Americans—the descendants of people first enslaved by European Americans (1619–1865), then "freed" to live as de jure second-class citizens (1865–1964), and now systematically denied economic opportunity and differentially incarcerated (1965–present)—proves this. An illustration of this is the fact that of the diseases reported to demonstrate a racial disparity in the tenth edition of *Robbins Basic Pathology*, published in 2017, the prevalence of twenty-two was higher in African Americans compared with only seven in European Americans.[2] Throughout this text and in several other works, I have demonstrated why these disparities are not simply the result of genetic differences between these groups.[3] Something else is going on, and part of that something was not understood until quite recently.

When I teach my students about the genome-to-phenotype pathway, I use the analogy of a murder mystery at a party. I point out that knowing the nucleotide sequence of an organism only tells you who was at the party. Gene expression tells you what the guests were doing. If you were trying to solve the murder, you might want to know if Colonel Mustard was in the study with the revolver when Mr. Boddy was killed. A few years back, my research group conducted an experiment to see if the bacterium *E. coli* could evolve resistance to excess iron in its culture medium and, if so, by what mechanisms.[4] This experiment was different from previous experimental evolution studies examining whether a bacterium could evolve resistance to a toxic substance such as an antibiotic or silver. In this case, iron is the key limiting element controlling bacterial growth. All cells, including ours, cannot function without iron as a critical cofactor with enzymes that catalyze key cellular functions. For this reason, bacteria excrete proteins called siderophores into their environment to sequester iron, which allows the iron to be taken in by cells. We found that *E. coli* could evolve resistance to excess iron, with four of our five experimental replicates carrying a mutation in the gene that encodes the Fe^{3+} dicitrate siderophore transport protein. This was a loss-of-function mutation that resulted in a reduction of the protein's ability to take up iron. You can think of this mutation as the smoking gun (or revolver) in the hands of the party guest (i.e., the Fe^{3+} dicitrate siderophore transport protein) who murdered Mr. Boddy. However, if we had concluded our investigation at this point, we would have missed other guests who also contributed to the murder. By using RNA sequencing technology, referred to as RNAseq, we were able to examine gene expression. The data showed that the iron-resistant *E. coli* populations also downregulated other genes associated with iron uptake and upregulated genes involved in protecting genes regulated by the ferric uptake regulator protein from oxidative stress. However, no genomic sequencing results could explain why this occurred, but it is likely that the changes in gene expression resulted from epigenetic changes. This is because bacteria have been shown to accumulate epigenetic modifications in response to stress and to pass them on to subsequent generations.[5]

From this example, we learn that even if we can demonstrate genetic differences between populations, we do not know the full story unless we understand the patterns of gene expression involved and how they produced the trait or condition of interest. This is well illustrated in a study of fruit flies that had been produced by experimental evolution differing in several life history characteristics, most notably development time and lifespan.[6] One of the fruit fly stocks (A stock) displayed accelerated development, greater reproduction in early life, overall lower stress resistance, and a shorter lifespan; a second stock showed slower development, lower reproduction in early life, higher stress resistance, and a longer lifespan (C stock). The transcriptome (i.e., the full range of messenger RNA expressed by an organism) of each stock of flies was examined on days 14 and 21 of their lifespans. On day 14, the mortality rates of the two stocks were not statistically significantly different from each other, but by day 21, the mortality rate of the A stock exceeded that of the C stock. On day 14, the RNA levels of protein-coding genes differed at 402 sites; by day 21, this number had grown to 482. Again, the protein-encoding genes were not telling the entire story. The study also found that on days 14 and 21, 136 and 246 noncoding RNAs were differentiated between the A and C stocks, respectively. Given the nature of the experimental design, this difference could not have occurred by chance. Thus, these noncoding RNAs were most likely interfering RNAs (noncoding RNAs involved in gene regulation), RNA interference being an epigenetic mechanism that plays a major role in gene expression.

EPIGENETIC MODIFICATION

Epigenetics refers to non-nucleotide-based changes in DNA that affect gene expression. All living things (i.e., viruses, bacteria, archaeans, and eukaryotes) use epigenetic tools to regulate their gene expression.[7] There are three types of epigenetic modification: microRNAs (miRNA), cytosine-phosphate-guanine (CpG) methylation, and histone modification. MiRNA and CpG methylation are found in all living things, and histone modification occurs mainly in eukaryotes (histone-like proteins are limited in bacteria and archaea). These three forms of epigenetic modification interact in particular instances of gene expression.[8]

It has been established that patterns of gene expression via epigenetic modification are associated with disease.[9] It is also known that some epigenetic modifications are inherited across generations. These two facts have particular importance in understanding how social subordination, a component of an organism's environment, can affect its biological functioning. In the context of structural racism, Arline Geronimus's weathering theory and Nancy Krieger's theory of ecosocial embodiment have played prominent roles in showing how social stressors contribute to physiological dysregulation.[10] Environmental stress can be transmitted across generations by the transmission of epigenetic modifications via germ-line cells, maternal experiences of stress that influence fetal epigenetic programming, and the experience of social stressors in both paternal and offspring generations. These forces can also combine with chronic exposure to adversity within a generation, which accelerates senescence and its associated physiological dysregulation—or weathering. These epigenetic modifications are thought to play a role in the threefold-higher rates of premature births and lower birth weights of African American infants compared with European American infants, as well as in the higher rates of hypertension, certain cancers, and shorter lifespans of African Americans compared with European Americans.[11]

Studies of epigenetic modification associated with disease are dominated by CpG methylation markers because they are the easiest to measure. This is because of the recent development of high-throughput chip-based methods that examine CpG methylation patterns across hundreds of thousands of sites. For example, Illumina's technology can estimate the methylation proportion for more than 850,000 sites in a given DNA sample.[12] However, Illumina sequencing is limited by its read length (about two hundred base pairs). Since the human genome comprises 3.3 billion base pairs, this means that it cannot determine linkage patterns in methylated sites along an entire chromosome. Humans have twenty-three chromosomes, and each chromosome has around 143 million base pairs. Thus, a sequencing technology that reads only two hundred base pairs at a time (with much of that DNA being short repeated sequences) cannot determine the positional relationship of all the nucleotide changes in that 143-million-nucleotide stretch, thus preventing the possibility of linkage analysis. But long-read sequencing technologies for CpG methylation have been developed. For example, Oxford Nanopore's sequencing technology can sequence CpG sites at a median length of eighty thousand base pairs.[13] This allows for a greater determination of potential linkage of methylated sites within the fragment of DNA sequenced.

The position of methylated sites in the genomes of organisms such as us matters. Our genomes contains stretches of nucleotides high in cytosines (C) and guanines (G). Areas made up of more than 55 percent C and G are called CpG islands if at least 65 percent have been methylated. The most important of the CpG islands are those located within two thousand bases of protein-coding genes. At these positions, methylation and demethylation patterns play a key role in gene expression. We know that 70 percent of gene promoters contain CpG islands.[14] Gene expression is suppressed by the methylation of CpG sites in the promoter region, which is located at the start of a gene. This is where the RNA polymerase enzyme binds to begin the transcription of the gene into messenger RNA. Messenger RNA carries the message that eventually produces the protein made from the gene in a process called translation. The suppression of gene expression occurs via the action of methyl-binding domain proteins, corepressor proteins, and histone deacetylases. Suppression can be undone by the action of methyl-cytosine dioxygenase, which removes the methyl-binding domain proteins, corepressor proteins, and the histone deacetylase complex by eliminating the methyl groups.

METHYLATION PATTERNS AND LIFESPAN

Biologically, the passage of chronological time is not the correct definition of senescence (i.e., aging) (see chapter 2). Our lifespan is divided into the developmental, reproductive, senescent, and late-life stages. During the first two stages, we do not age. Aging begins after our net future expected reproduction has reached or is very close to zero. Progression through life span stages can be measured via biomarkers such as methylation levels in DNA. Thus the amount of methylation across the genome can be used to effectively determine an individual's biological, as opposed to chronological, age.[15] This makes sense because it is well known that gene expression in key maintenance-associated systems declines with age.[16] As we age, mitochondrial proteins, protein synthesis, and growth factor signaling are downregulated; the immune system, gene regulation, and messenger RNA processing become dysregulated; and we experience constitutive responses to stress and DNA damage. Constitutive defenses are those that are "turned on" all the time, whereas inducible defenses are turned on only to address a specific need, such as fighting infection.

Owing to the population genetic mechanisms of aging (see chapter 2) and differences in environmental exposures, people differ in the onset and rate of senescence. Further, given that most, or possibly all, protein-coding genes expressed in the human genome contribute to senescence, it is highly likely that there is more variation in lifespan within populations than between them. Using data from the US National Vital Statistics 2015 life table for Black and white populations, I computed mean lifespans of 76.4 years for whites and 73 years for Blacks.[17] The mean difference between groups was 3.4 years. However, the variance in lifespan for each group was 260 and 337 years, respectively. Thus, the variances were 76.5 and 99 times the mean difference for whites and Blacks, respectively. These findings demonstrate that within-group lifespan variance is much greater than between-groups variance in lifespan. This basic fact of biology is not understood by all.

For example, a 2016 survey of University of Virginia medical students showed that 33.3, 38.9, 20.3, and 50 percent of first-year students, second-year students, third-year students, and residents, respectively, believed that Blacks aged more slowly than whites.[18] One has to wonder what "evidence" they used to come to this conclusion. My guess is that they were thinking of skin wrinkling and did not know that darker skin does a better job than lighter skin of protecting itself from UV damage.

However, we know that rates of mean age-specific morbidity (i.e., sickness) and mortality (i.e., death) are higher in Blacks than in whites for all periods of American history.[19] Further, methylation patterns across the genome (not just in the skin) demonstrate that Blacks age more quickly in the United States than whites. In a study of more than four hundred individuals examining age-specific cellular pathways associated with aging, Black participants were found to have 4,930 compared to only 469 for white participants. The higher number for Blacks was calculated as an increase in biological age of about two years.[20] However, methylation patterns associated with age-specific diseases do not seem to be consistent with socially defined race. In another study using the same sample of people, researchers found that differential patterns of hypo- and hyper-methylated genes were associated with a higher prevalence of metabolic syndrome in Blacks (see chapter 3).[21] Metabolic syndrome is defined by central obesity (based on population-specific criteria) and any two of the following: increased triglycerides, reduced high-density lipoprotein (HDL) cholesterol, hypertension, and elevated fasting plasma glucose or diagnosed diabetes. However, data indicated that Blacks had lower levels of methylation in immune system genes compared to whites, indicating a slower decline of immune function in Blacks. This observation is consistent with earlier observations of longer telomere lengths in leukocytes (white blood cells, crucial to immune function) with age in Blacks compared to whites.[22] Telomeres are the end regions of chromosomes, and their length shortens with the number of cell divisions that occur in eukaryotes; thus, telomere length is used as a biomarker of aging. Data like this also underscore the lack of concordance between supposed genetic differences and observed disease and life history phenotypes. The supposed slower decline of immune function predicted from these studies is in opposition to the greater increase in age-associated infectious diseases and cancers in Blacks compared to whites in America. This indicates that environmental factors also influence the observed differences.

ENVIRONMENTAL CONTRIBUTORS TO EPIGENETIC CHANGE

Abundant evidence has demonstrated that epigenetic programming in animals is passed on from generation to generation, particularly in the form of maternal effects. This is one of the reasons that, in all experimental evolution work on aging, we require control and treatment populations to undergo two generations of common environmental conditions before measuring any phenotypic effects. Allowing for two generations reduces differences in maternal effects that could interfere with the assessment of the physiological results attributed to the experimental selection to which the studied organisms, often fruit flies, are exposed.[23] The fact that socially defined races of humans have never shared common environments also complicates the assessment of genetic contributions to health disparities or other physiological conditions measured between groups.

During fertilization, sperm cells generally carry high amounts of DNA methylation across the genome, whereas egg cells generally carry a low load.[24] The patterns of methylation in sperm and egg cells differ, and after fertilization the paternal genome experiences a rapid decline in methylation. Next, a wave of de novo methylation occurs in the late-preimplantation embryo that restores methylation to levels similar to those observed in adult somatic cells.[25] Methylation continues across the lifespan, and methylation levels are associated with various psychosocial stressors. It is well known that psychosocial stressors in early life, such as prenatal exposure to intimate partner violence, war-related stress, and child abuse affect methylation levels in the NR3C1 gene.[26] This gene encodes the glucocorticoid receptor that regulates the function of the hypothalamus–pituitary–adrenal (HPA) axis. The HPA axis begins its development during gestation and plays a critical role in stress response. A study of intergenerational trauma using data from the war-torn region of the Democratic Republic of the Congo and from a database of Canadian mothers found that methylation of genes such as BDNF (brain-derived neurotrophic factor), CRH (corticotrophin-releasing hormone), CRHBP (corticotrophin-releasing hormone-binding protein), FKBPF (responsible for immunoregulation and basic cellular processes), and IGF1 (insulin-like growth factor 1) results from early-life trauma.[27] It is also known that the degree of methylation of these genes is associated with the severity of trauma experienced during childhood.[28] On the flip side, research shows that emotional support and prosocial ties with parents, peers, partners, and mentors are inversely associated with methylation. An example of this was found in a study of the *OXTR* gene (which encodes the oxytocin receptor) in young Black men.[29] The significance of this study cannot be understated given that oxytocin is involved in the ability to feel love and empathy. Findings like this demonstrate that prosocial environments are more likely to produce human beings capable of empathy than are stressful environments.

Dozens of studies have now been published on the impact of adverse environmental effects on epigenetic modification, mainly methylation.[30] Risk factors include maternal and prenatal adversity, childhood adversity, adult psychosocial stress, lower socioeconomic status, racism and discrimination, neighborhood social environment, sexual assault, and exposure to war or criminal violence. These stressors have been associated with increased methylation in at least 160 human genes. We also know that these stressors are differentially associated with socially defined race in the United States. For example, maternal experiences of adversity may play a role in preterm birth, and birth weight is a strong predictor of infant health and of disease in later life. Data has shown that a similar birth weight distribution occurs among African women born in Africa and European American women, whereas the distribution among African American women is statistically significantly lower.[31] Birth weight is a function of gestation period, with prematurely born infants typically being of statistically significantly lower weight than full-term infants. One study examined the methylation patterns in genetic variants associated with preterm birth in Black and non-Black mothers. The researchers found that methylation patterns at three CpG sites in the *TNFAIP8* (TNF alpha-induced protein 8) gene, which plays a role in apoptosis (programmed cell death), and the *PON1* (paraoxonase 1) gene, which is involved in breaking down lactones and esters, were statistically significantly different between Black and non-Black infants.[32] Maternal stress has also been shown to be associated with increased methylation in gene regulatory sequences in offspring. Differential methylation patterns between Blacks and whites have also been found to play a role in breast, colon, and prostate cancer predisposition.[33]

Studies have also shown how racial discrimination affects cognitive and emotional function. Repeated exposure to racial discrimination has been directly connected to a greater incidence of brain health disorders.[34] And the frequency of discriminatory events is associated with a greater prevalence and severity of brain health disorders such as post-traumatic stress syndrome and major depressive disorder. Thus, the experience of racial discrimination may contribute to the US Black population's two-fold greater probability of developing Alzheimer's disease comparted to the US white population.[35] One study examined the impact of post-traumatic stress syndrome resulting from racial discrimination in Black women (with a mean age of 38.5 years), with aspects of brain connectivity and epigenetic modifications calculated from leukocytes. The study found that those who had experienced greater racial discrimination had greater locus coeruleus resting-state brain connectivity to the bilateral precuneus region of the brain, a region involved in reliving past events. The authors also found a statistically significant correlation between this neural connection and epigenetic age, or DNA methylation age acceleration (DMAA), calculated using a DMAA index referred to as the Horvath clock.[36] The Horvath clock is an estimation of biological as opposed to chronological age based on the amount of CpG methylation. This finding is yet another powerful illustration of how racial discrimination harms Black people.

In addition to social aspects of the environment, physical exposures play a role in altering epigenetic profiles. Lead exposure is common and has a cumulative effect on DNA methylation.[37] Lead is a divalent cation, which allows it to enter cells via calcium channels. Inside the cell, lead causes oxidative stress by generating free radicals that react with proteins and nucleic acids, which can create nucleotide-based changes—mutations—as well as epigenetic modifications. Lead has also been shown to react with *DNMT* enzyme complexes, which play a critical role in methylation.

High levels of lead in the maternal body have been associated with the hypomethylation of *COL1A2* (collagen type 1 alpha 2) and *ROCK1* (Rho-associated coiled-coil-containing protein kinase 1). Hypomethylation of the former is associated with preterm birth and hypomethylation of the latter with birth defects. Lead has also been associated with hypermethylation of the *PLAG1* (zinc finger pleomorphic adenoma gene 1), *HYMAI* (which encodes a noncoding RNA), *IGF2* (insulin growth factor 2), and *H19* (which encodes a long noncoding RNA that acts as a tumor suppressor) genes. Hypermethylation of these four genes is associated with fetal growth restriction.

Lead exposure is differentially experienced by socially defined race. The Third National Health and Nutrition Examination Survey found close to three times the level of lead in Black children compared to white children between 1999 and 2002.[38] Lead exposure is also associated with residential segregation in the United States. And the situation is not getting better. For example, between 1999 and 2015 in North Carolina, there was a 50 percent increase in residential segregation. One study found that for one standard deviation increase in residential segregation, blood lead levels increased by 2.86 and 2.44 percent, respectively, in Black and white children.[39]

Finally, given the mechanism by which lead causes epigenetic changes, we should expect that other heavy metals and organic or metal compounds would cause similar effects. Indeed, evidence shows that other heavy metals such as cadmium and mercury and organic chemicals such as per- and polyfluoroalkyl substances (PFAS) also cause alterations in epigenetic gene regulation.[40] Exposure to such metals and compounds are also differentially experienced by socially defined race, with Black and Brown people receiving more exposure via mechanisms such as air pollution and living in proximity to toxic waste sites.[41]

THE EPIGENOMICS OF THE BROKEN HEART

Cardiovascular (heart) disease (CVD) is now the leading late-age cause of mortality in the United States, having taken over first spot from infectious disease in the middle of the twentieth century. Unsurprisingly, a pronounced health disparity in CVD mortality existed between Blacks in whites throughout the twentieth century and continues to exist today. Figure 8.1 shows the

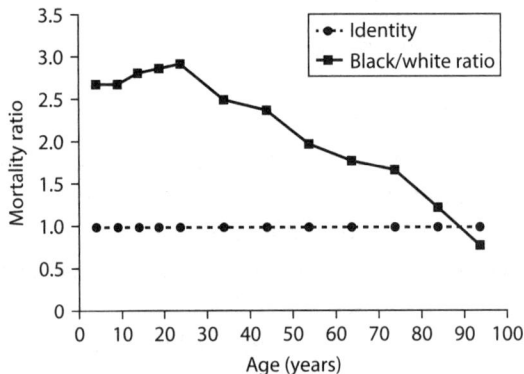

FIGURE 8.1. The age-specific mortality ratio for cardiovascular disease in Blacks and whites in the United States, 2021 *Source:* Adapted and updated from S. C. Curtin et al., "Deaths: Leading Causes for 2021," *National Vital Statistics Reports* 73, no. 4 (2024), https://www.cdc.gov/nchs/data/nvsr/nvsr73/nvsr73-04.pdf.

age-specific mortality ratio for CVD in Blacks and whites in the United States for 2021.

This figure shows that Black mortality greatly exceeds white mortality at all ages except for the highest age category of more than eighty-five years, a pattern that has persisted since the early twentieth century.[42] As CVD is a disease of both homeostasis and maintenance, it is extremely rare at young ages (occurring in fewer than twenty individuals per one hundred thousand in Blacks and eight per one hundred thousand in whites below the age of thirty-four years). However, the rate of CVD mortality increases exponentially after the age of fifty years, as expected of diseases of maintenance. It is the number-one cause of mortality for Blacks between the ages of forty-four and fifty-four years and for whites between the ages of seventy-four and eighty-four years.

The prevalence of CVD is profoundly influenced by evolutionary mismatch. The environments of all modern human populations are mismatched relative to those of our ancestral hunter-gatherers, which featured much greater daily activity and a diet lower in calories.[43] The hominid lineage (i.e., the evolutionary group of "great apes") produced omnivorous hunter-gatherer species. Our species evolved behaviors that rewarded the acquisition of high-calorie, sweet, and fatty foods as such a diet would have improved the likelihood of survival and reproduction in pre-agricultural populations. But the development of agriculture made possible the production of food in excess, and this occurred only very recently in the history of human evolution, about ten thousand years ago or less.[44] Indeed, for populations living in industrialized nations, an excess of food did not become available until well after the Industrial Revolution of the eighteenth century.[45]

The pleasure centers in the brain that respond to high-calorie, sweet, and fatty foods are also those that are activated by concentrated drugs, gambling, and sexual activity.[46] Thus, it is not by chance that the rise of these problems in industrialized societies coincided with increases in the means of providing addictive substances to their populations as they became more industrialized and now more technologically advanced (e.g., highly concentrated drugs, both legal and illegal; alcohol and tobacco; online gambling and sports betting; ultra-processed foods and food additives like high-fructose corn syrup).

Populations of societies that have long been industrialized experience higher rates of CVD than those who have only more recently become industrialized. For example, between 1951 and 1956, 33 percent of American men aged seventy to seventy-nine years showed evidence of myocardial infarction (heart attack) at autopsy, compared to 0 percent of Ugandan men.[47] Rates of CVD have also greatly increased in Asia and Africa as a result of economic changes and rapid urbanization, respectively.[48] It has been argued that 90 percent of the global burden of myocardial infarction can be explained by apolipoprotein B:A ratio, smoking, diabetes, hypertension, abdominal obesity, poor diet, low physical activity, and psychosocial stress.

These risk factors illustrate that CVD is a complex phenotype with both genetic and environmental contributors, as shown by a recent genome-wide association (GWAS) study that found the polygenic risk score for South Asians included more than six million common genetic variants.[49] In contrast to this kind of analysis, a recent study of the prevalence of hereditary transthyretin (TTR) amyloid cardiomyopathy has been associated with the dominant genetic variant V122I (valine-to-isoleucine substitution at position 122 of the protein).[50] Amyloid cardiomyopathy is a form of restrictive cardiomyopathy (heart disease) characterized by a decrease in ventricular functioning during diastole contraction. In this case, the reduced functioning results from the deposition of extracellular proteins that tend to form insoluble beta-pleated sheets, which impairs the heart muscle's ability to contract.[51]

The presence of the V122I variant in the *TTR* gene that encodes the transthyretin protein can result in a protein misfolding that allows the accumulation of insoluble, extracellular amyloid fibrils in the myocardium (the thick middle layer of the heart). To evaluate the role of this variant in hereditary TTR amyloid cardiomyopathy, researchers assessed genomic data from the Penn Medicine BioBank and the BioMe BioBank for more than ninety thousand patients and found that 92 of 237 TTR V122I variant carriers experienced heart failure after the age of sixty-five years). The researchers computed that the presence of this variant increased the odds ratio of heart failure by 1.7 to 1.8.

This variant is of interest with regard to the disparity in CVD between Blacks and whites because of the higher prevalence of CVD in populations of African descent. The V122I variant is not found in Eastern Hemisphere populations outside West Africa, and not all West African populations show the variant. But because of its origin in West Africa, the variant is found in Western Hemisphere populations with a larger degree of African ancestry, such as African Americans, African Caribbeans, and Latin Americans. It is also observed at low frequencies in some European-descended and Indigenous American populations; here, it is most likely the result of African admixture into these groups. However, it is clear from this study that the V122I variant contributes only slightly to the disparity in CVD rates between Black and white populations. Of the 9,694 individuals socially defined as Black or Hispanic in this study, only 237 where carriers of the V122I variant (meaning these populations had a carrier frequency of only 0.024). The mortality rate ratio for Black people aged sixty-four to seventy-four years ranged from 1.22 to 1.78 times higher than white people of the same age. The presence of this variant in only about 2 percent of Black people cannot account for such a huge disparity.

Epigenetic markers influenced by environmental factors have been shown to play a major role in coronary heart disease (CHD).[52] By 2020, GWAS studies had identified more than 150 single-nucleotide polymorphisms (SNPs) associated with coronary heart disease (CHD).[53] Unsurprisingly, these were located in genes related to lipid metabolism, inflammation, transcriptional regulation, blood pressure, cell proliferation, neovascularization angiogenesis, nitric oxide signaling, and vascular remodeling. Yet these SNPs accounted for only about 10 percent of the heritability (h^2) of CHD (remember that h^2 is a measure of the genetic contribution of a complex trait).[54] This finding suggested that other factors, such as epigenetic modifications, must contribute to the "missing heritability" of CVD.

In 2019, a blood leukocyte DNA methylation study of more than eleven thousand people was conducted to examine epigenetic contributions to myocardial infarction and coronary artery disease.[55] The data came from nine groups involved in CVD studies from the United States and Europe. The data for Black individuals came from the Atherosclerosis Risk in Community (ARIC) Study, whose Black cohorts lived in Jackson, Mississippi, and Forsyth County, North Carolina. The entire sample of the 2019 study had a mean age of about sixty-four years, 67 percent were female, and 35 percent were Black. Of the 442,192 CpG methylation sites examined, thirty were found to be associated with current or future coronary artery disease, and another twenty-nine were associated with myocardial infarction; both sets displayed association probabilities between 10^{-8} to 10^{-6}. Remember that in GWAS studies, the gold standard for statistical significance is 10^{-8} because GWAS studies typically assess millions of sites. At this level of statistical significance, we would expect zero false discoveries examining 442,192 sites.

This is equivalent to a type II statistical error which means accepting a null hypothesis when it is actually false, in this case claiming the genetic variant contributes to the condition, when it does not. Here, 10^{-6} also provides about zero false discoveries ($442{,}192 \times 10^{-6} = 0.442$, which is closer to 0 than to 1).

The researchers examined the significant CpG sites associated with coronary artery disease and found that eleven of fifty-two were differentiated by socially defined race. This is not to be unexpected since African Americans have both African and European ancestry. Some of the sites associated with coronary artery disease are ancient, meaning that methylation at those sites was occurring before migration out of Africa began; the eleven differentiated sites would have become differentiated after gene flow between Africa and Europe was reduced by geographic distance. Also, because the African Americans in this study contained on average 16 percent European ancestry, many of their CpG sites would have derived from their European ancestry, not their African ancestry. Further, genetic linkage between genes on chromosomes differs by continental origin. Because the human species originated in Africa and because of a crossing-over process known as meiosis that occurs across generations, African linkage blocks are smaller than those of Europeans. This is why many GWAS results in African and European populations do not match.[56]

Further studies of methylation associated with CVD called epigenome-wide association (EWAS) studies have examined about 450,000 CpG sites, mostly in European populations.[57] EWAS studies replicate many of the genetic loci described earlier but include at least seventy additional sites, such as ZBTB12 (zinc finger and BTB domain containing 12), SLC9A1 (solute carrier family 9, member A1), SLC1A5 (solute carrier family 1, member 5), TNRC6C (trinucleotide repeat-containing adapter 6C), and TSSC1 (tumor-suppressing subtransferable candidate 1). Because these genes contain multiple methylation sites, it is unsurprising that one study identified at least 143 CpG positions with impacts on CVD and myocardial infarction. In addition, at least fifteen interfering RNAs have been associated with CVD.[58] These findings conclusively demonstrate that the various types of CVD are complex traits influenced by genetic, epigenetic, and environmental effects.

The modern data presents a compelling argument for how patterns of epigenetic modification caused by both physical and social differences driven by structural racism play an important role in the health and mortality profiles of socially defined races in the United States. Because CVD must occur eventually because it is a disease of maintenance, it is by no means easy to predict when the heart will get broken. Nor are there any intrinsic genetic reasons for certain socially defined racial groups such as African Americans to experience differential rates of morbidity and mortality from CVD. Additional research is needed to quantify just how much of a role the various factors that contribute to CVD (i.e., genetics, epigenetics, the environment, and chance) play in the observed differentials, but what is clear is that improving the social and physical environments of those differentially affected—that is, African Americans—would help reverse the problem. Yet we also know that epigenetic effects are transmitted across generations, so if we want to see a reduction in differential morbidity and mortality rates any time soon, we must begin to dismantle the structural inequalities that exist in this nation immediately.

Chapter Nine

HOW ALGORITHMS CAN HURT

Algorithms are defined as processes or rules to be followed in calculations or other problem-solving operations, especially by computers. They work pretty well if there is a strong functional relationship between the quantities in the calculation. For example, it is relatively easy to convert temperature on the Fahrenheit scale to Celsius: $C = [(F - 32)/1.8]$. So, we would compute 100°F as follows:

$$C = [(100 - 32)/1.8]$$
$$C = [(64)/1.8]$$
$$C = 35.5°$$

If we use the algorithm over and over again for different values (in a process known as iterative calculation), we can better see the relationship between the two temperature scales (figure 9.1). The relationship is linear, and if you know what X (temperature in Celsius) is, then you automatically know what Y (temperature in Fahrenheit) is.

But the problem is far more difficult if variability is built into the equation. Instead of a fixed slope of 1.8, as in figure 9.1, let's allow the slope to vary randomly from 1.0 to 2.0 (figure 9.2).

Now the results will vary depending on which randomly chosen value for the slope was used to compute the value of temperature in Celsius. In some cases, the new values will be close to those shown in figure 9.1, but in many

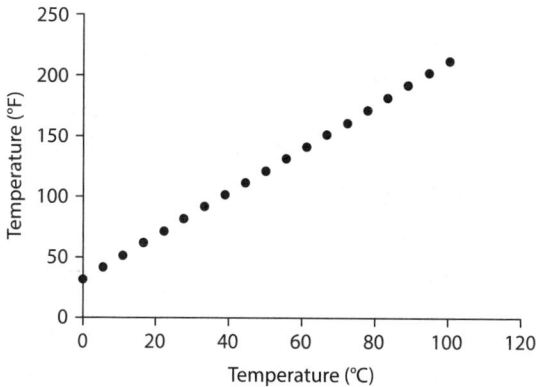

FIGURE 9.1. Conversion between the Celsius and Fahrenheit temperature scales

cases, the new values will be very different. Further, if we run the calculation again with a new set of randomly chosen values, the overall shape of the curve would be similar, but the individual points would vary. This simple example illustrates the inherent problem of using algorithms to compute values for biological organisms. Variation is a fundamental aspect of biology. The variation of the biological trait in question is directly related to the genetic complexity associated with determining the trait. The more genetic, environmental, and chance factors involved, the more unpredictable the outcome will be. Thus, there is variation both between and within human populations. Further, the use of standard algorithms to compute population

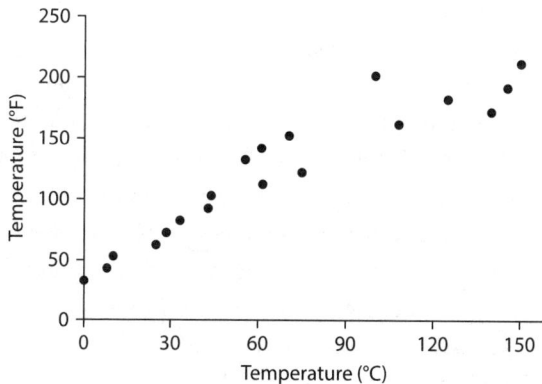

FIGURE 9.2. Conversion between the Celsius and Fahrenheit temperature scales with randomness

differences—that is, differences between socially defined racial groups—in complex traits such as body weight, bone density, kidney function, and lung function are flawed at the root. In some cases, the flaws are just a nuisance, but in other cases, they can cause significant harm. It is no accident that the historical harm caused by the use of medical algorithms has always been visited on socially subordinated groups of people.

BIOLOGICAL VARIATION WITHIN AND BETWEEN GROUPS

More than eighty years ago, field biologists recognized that trait variation within species occurred in a graded fashion. Julian Huxley coined the term *cline* to describe gradients in measurable physical traits.[1] It was also noticed around this time that clines in the various physical characters of organisms, including humans, did not always correlate with one another. This notion led Huxley to be one of the first biologists to object to the use of *race* as an adequate term to describe human variation.[2] By 1962, the University of Michigan biological anthropologist Frank Livingstone had stated that there were no human races, only clines.[3] C. Loring Brace would take this idea further by pointing out that the analysis of human traits required the analysis of the selection pressures influencing each physical trait separately.[4] This is well illustrated by examining the distribution of physical traits such as skin color, hair type, hair color, tooth size and shape, disease resistance adaptations (such as the sickle cell allele, discussed in chapter 6), and blood type.[5] These traits do not correlate with one another because each is acted on by the evolutionary forces of selection and genetic drift in different ways. For example, a strong north–south gradient exists in skin color, and thus in the alleles associated with skin color, in Eastern Hemisphere populations from the tropics to the Arctic (figure 9.3).

Here, I am referring to the populations that settled in these regions during ancient human migrations (not recent migrations, such as those of Europeans to Africa during the colonial period or of Africans to Europe in the present). However, there is no north–south gradient in the sickle cell allele (Hb_S) or in alleles associated with adaptation to high altitude because the frequency of these traits is determined, respectively, by the presence or absence of malaria and the presence or absence of high mountains. Thus, we find both dark- and light-skinned people with and without Hb_S and with and without high-altitude adaptations. The lack of correlation between physical traits is called the principle of discordance.[6]

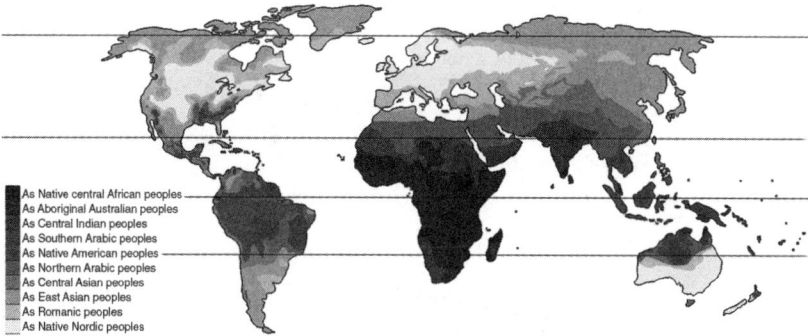

FIGURE 9.3. Human skin color map, twenty-first century *Source*: "Human Skin Color by the 21st Century. Native People Data by Renato Biasutti Plus Data from 19th and 20th Centuries' Migrations from National Censuses," Wikimedia Commons, uploaded February 17, 2019, https://commons.wikimedia.org/w/index.php?search=Biasutti+skin+color&title=Special:MediaSearch&go=Go&type=image.

Indeed, if you try to use human physical traits to compute trees of evolutionary relatedness, you will come to the wrong conclusions. The eminent anthropologist Luigi Luca Cavalli-Sforza and the biostatistician A. W. F. Edwards did just that in a 1964 paper in which they used general anthropometric characters, including skin color and whole-body attributes, to draw such trees.[7] The first split in the tree separated groups with darker skin (Papua New Guineans, Indigenous Australians, sub-Saharan Bantu-speaking people, Pygmies, and Bushmen) from those with lighter skin (Swedish, French, Eskimo, North American Indian, Japanese, Chinese, South American Indian, Ainu, Maori, and Polynesian groups). If you are familiar with human evolution, you will recognize that this classification is incorrect as sub-Saharan African populations are more closely related to Europeans than to Indigenous Australians or Papua New Guineans. The fallacy of this categorization is further revealed in the branching pattern of the lighter-skinned populations, which grouped Swedes, French people, Eskimo, and North American Indians as one major group and Japanese, Chinese, South American Indians, Ainu, Maori, and Polynesians as another. From both fossil and genetic evidence, we know that North and South American Indians are more closely related to each other than to the other groups they are linked to in this tree.[8] Thus, we cannot use physical traits to divide people into groups that conform with the known evolutionary history of our species. This creates a problem for the use of any algorithm based on specific physical traits because attributes like body type and bone density vary both between and within population groups.

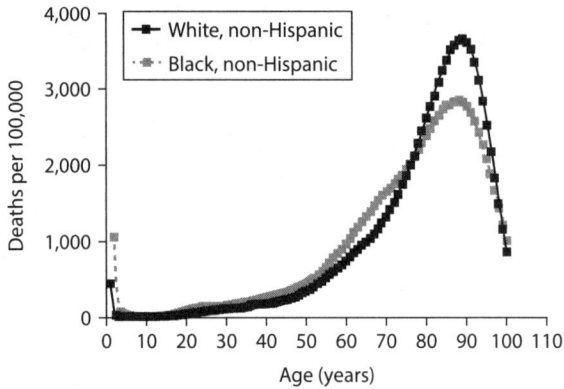

FIGURE 9.4. Life expectancy for Black and white Americans, 2019

Within-group variation is particularly problematic for the accuracy of medical algorithms. Racialized algorithms operate by using a mean difference between groups; however, traits such as lung function, bone density, cognitive function, blood pressure, pharmacokinetic response (i.e., how the body metabolizes a drug), and birth weight are all quantitative traits. This means that the traits are variable within populations, often described by the normal statistical distribution (also called the bell curve). This means that while one can compute an average value for a trait, many people will fall significantly above or below the mean depending on how variable the trait is. Further, if you are comparing a quantitative trait between groups, even if there is a statistically significant difference between the means, depending on the variance of the trait, there will still be substantial overlap between the distributions, meaning that individuals from both groups will display the trait. Figure 9.4 shows life expectancy for Black and white Americans in 2019. While there is a statistically significant difference between groups, with Blacks tending to die at younger ages than whites, substantial numbers of both groups experienced all lifespans.

MEASURING VARIATION

The advent of wearable technology has revolutionized our ability to collect physiological data from humans. A recent study conducted in Ann Arbor, Michigan, involved providing 6,454 participants an Apple Watch (series 3 or 4), an Omron Evolv wireless blood pressure monitor, and the MyDataHelps smartphone app to record data.[9] The participants wore the blood pressure monitor for twelve or more hours per day while conducting their normal daily and weekly tasks. The researchers measured their heart rate, step count, and distance walked. Data was disaggregated by socially defined race: white (n = 3,657), Black (n = 1,094), Asian (n = 1,090), and other (n = 612). In individuals not undergoing treatment for hypertension, the mean daily systolic blood pressure was as follows: white, 121 (standard deviation [SD], +/−10); Black, 122 (SD, +/−10); Asian, 118 (SD, +/−9), and other, 118 (SD, +/−9). These differences are not statistically significantly different, meaning that the distributions overlapped such that it would been impossible to associate socially defined race with a particular systolic blood pressure measurement. The diastolic blood pressure measurements showed the same pattern: white, 76 (SD, +/−7); Black, 77 (SD, +/−8); Asian, 76 (SD, +/−7); and other, 75 (+/−7). Similar patterns were seen by socially defined race for individuals receiving treatment for hypertension (systolic pressure, 129–127 [SD, +/−8−10]). Yet despite the one-point mean difference in the blood pressure measurements (which was statistically significant at $p < 0.005$), the authors still felt compelled to state, "Black participants had the highest systolic and diastolic blood pressures of any race."[10] This statistical difference resulted from the very large number of individuals measured (n = 4,751). However, one would have a difficult time making the case that a one-point difference in systolic and diastolic blood pressure has any clinical value in predicting whether a given patient will have a blood pressure value due to their socially defined race. With data this similar, one could not determine a person's socially defined race by their blood pressure measurements or vice versa. The authors' decision to state that Black participants had the highest blood pressure speaks to the ongoing implicit racial bias in biomedical research.

Implicit bias in biomedical research results primarily from the socially defined categories used by researchers. The ancestry of those lumped into the Black category was not described in this study. Were they African American (i.e., descendants of enslaved people in America), African Caribbean, West African (e.g., Nigerians), or East African (e.g., Kenyans)? The typological characterization of people with African descent ignores the facts that Africans show the greatest amount of genetic diversity of all groups of humans on the planet and that the continent of Africa has eight climatic zones to which human populations adapted during the three hundred thousand years our species has existed. With the growing emigration of people from African nations, the diversity within the African diaspora cannot be ignored in medical research.[11] The diversity of the Black population must be considered because African Americans have high amounts of European ancestry (about 16 percent on average), whereas East, South, and West Africans generally have none. But bias toward and typological thinking about Black people often find their way into algorithms designed to provide patient care.[12]

PULMONARY FUNCTION

Thomas Jefferson was the first person to claim that there were differences in lung capacity between Blacks and whites in the United States.[13] The idea was latter amplified by Samuel Cartwright, who argued in the 1800s that there was a 20 percent deficiency in Black lung capacity. Cartwright used this notion to buttress the system of American slavery by arguing that enforced labor would *improve* Black lung function. Of course, Cartwright did not consider that it might have been the deprivations created by the institution of slavery that were responsible for the decreased lung capacity of enslaved people. Nor were any comparative measurements taken of free people of African descent in the United States or of those from West Africa. Without such measurements for comparison, it would have been impossible to claim that decreased lung function was a racial trait.

Both Jefferson and Cartwright argued for an innate racial difference in the context of special creationism, a belief system purporting that God created Blacks to be innately inferior to whites in a variety of traits, not just lung function.[14] In this system of racial classification, the notion that individuals within "races" display variability in physical characteristics was not understood. For example, Jefferson and Cartwright would have considered individuals from the Simien Plateau in Northern Ethiopia "Negro." Yet these people have superior lung capacity compared with lowland populations (both European and African). Individuals living at the Simien Plateau are able to maintain the same levels of oxygen saturation of arterial blood and hemoglobin as Ethiopians living at sea level. Thus, these populations do not respond to hypoxic (low-oxygen) stress with erythrocytosis (an increase in the number of red blood cells in the blood), and they do not suffer from arterial hypoxemia (an abnormally low concentration of oxygen in the blood). Recent work suggests that these populations show increased concentrations of nitric oxide and cyclic guanosine monophosphate, suggesting that adaptation occurs via vasodilation (the widening of blood vessels).[15] In addition, their cerebral circulation is sensitive to nitric oxide and carbon dioxide, which increase cerebral blood flow and oxygen delivery to the brain. These adaptations have contributed to the dominance of long-distance runners from Ethiopia and Kenya in international competition.

The notion of the innateness of inferior pulmonary function in Blacks went unchallenged into the twenty-first century. In 2012, the Global Lung Function Initiative published race-corrected equations for whites, African Americans, Northeast Asians, Southeast Asians, and people of other races or mixed race. These correction factors were derived from African Americans living in the United States, and no systematic study of pulmonary function in Black populations across Africa, the Caribbean, or South America was conducted.[16] Yet the authors should have realized that their reasoning was deeply flawed because modern biology recognizes that the genetic basis of all phenotypes evolved and all phenotypes are expressed in the context of people's environments. The factors known to contribute to "normal" lung function are age, gender, body composition, and ethnicity.[17] Yet ethnicity is most likely a proxy for other unmeasured aspects of biological and environmental variation affecting lung function. Pulmonary function clearly differs between high- and low-altitude populations. High-altitude populations display adaptation to the lower amounts of oxygen at high elevations. In contrast, low-altitude populations are often exposed differentially to air pollution. But the idea that entire socially defined races should differ in pulmonary function does not make any sense. Known factors that negatively affect pulmonary function, which also differ between socially defined races include exposure to pesticides and lead, smoking status (and type of cigarettes used), childhood respiratory illnesses (infectious and autoimmune), obesity, and structural racism in the form of lack of access to high-quality primary care, food deserts in poor neighborhoods, high rates of incarceration, and stress resulting from racial subordination.[18]

Finally, recent studies of race correction in spirometry (the measure of lung function) have been shown to lead to misdiagnosis or misclassification of medical diagnosis in asthma and chronic obstructive pulmonary disease.[19] Such studies have caused the US House Committee on Ways & Means to publish a report calling for the end of the misuse of race in clinical decision support tools, including pulmonary function tests.[20] The Global Lung Function Initiative has since released a new equation that does not use race correction. A study of 8,431 Black and white Americans found that the new equation increased the number of Black individuals identified as having a restrictive ventilatory impairment by 10.7 percent and reduced the number of white individuals with such a diagnosis by 4.6 percent.[21]

BONE DENSITY

The FRAX algorithm is used to measure the risk of osteoporosis-related fractures by race. This tool was developed to predict an individual's ten-year probability of major osteoporotic fracture (composite of hip, humerus, forearm, and clinical vertebral fractures) and hip fracture from their clinical risk factors.[22] The FRAX tool is calibrated to a target population using population-specific fracture and mortality data, and more than seventy countries use FRAX tools. The United States uses four calculators of bone density defined by socially defined race and ethnicity: white ("Caucasian"), Black, Asian, and Hispanic. White, Black, and Asian are socially defined races, whereas *Hispanic* refers to ethnicity. This term is particularly useless when attempting to predict bone density because *Hispanic* refers only to whether someone speaks Spanish as their primary language. This means that people with varying amounts of African, European, and Indigenous American ancestry are all lumped into this category. It also means that individuals with similar amounts of these ancestries from similar parts of the world are not included in this group, such as Brazilians (who speak Portuguese) and Haitians (who speak French). The white calculator was calibrated directly using fracture data; nonwhite calculators incorporated calibration multipliers (for Blacks, 0.43 for women and 0.53 for men; for Asians, 0.50 for women and 0.64 for men; for Hispanics, 0.53 for women and 0.58 for men). This means that likelihood of fracture occurring is calculated for non-whites by multiplying the calibration multiplier figure.[23]

The use of race correction in predicting osteoporosis risk originated from a study conducted in 1960.[24] It found that peak bone mass density was greater in Blacks than whites. The Black population was sampled from individuals descended from enslaved people in the United States. Yet we know that the ancestry of this group is not representative of all Africans. African American ancestry includes contributions from West and Central Africa (about 84 percent on average) and Northwestern Europe (about 16 percent on average).[25] The individuals described as white in this study were primarily from Western and Northern Europe. This group has more than 98 percent European ancestry, with 25 to 55 percent British or Irish ancestry and

5 to 20 percent Scandinavian.[26] The lack of sampling across human populations means that the findings of this study cannot be used to make a general statement about bone density in either African or European populations. As mentioned, Africans display the greatest genetic variation of all groups in our species. Further, bone density is determined by several genetic and environmental factors, including nutrition (e.g., calcium and vitamin D intake), sun exposure (i.e., vitamin D intake), stress (e.g., cortisol levels), hormone levels (e.g., estrogen, parathyroid hormone, insulin), and growth factors (e.g., insulin-like growth factor 1 [IGF1]), as well as body mass index, smoking status, alcohol consumption, physical activity level, and long-term use of medications such as glucocorticoids.[27] We also know that epigenetic modifications play crucial roles in osteogenic differentiation, osteogenesis, bone remodeling, and other bone-related metabolic processes.[28] The interaction of genetic, epigenetic, and environmental factors guarantees that human populations are variable across physiological phenotypes, including bone density. For example, many East African populations have lower bone density than Western and Northern European populations.[29] The census categories used in the United States define a person as Black if they have any detectable African ancestry, including from East African nations.[30]

Given that we have no comprehensive survey of the bone densities of populations across the globe and that populations cannot be unambiguously grouped into biological races, the idea of race correction for bone density is misleading. Indeed, a recent study found that using a population-based FRAX calculator, as opposed to the existing racial and ethnic FRAX calculators, would reduce differences in treatment qualification and ultimately enhance equity and access to osteoporosis treatment.[31]

KIDNEY FUNCTION

The kidneys function to regulate water and inorganic ion balance and to remove metabolic waste products and foreign chemicals from the blood to be excreted in urine. They also add glucose to the bloodstream via gluconeogenesis (the process of making glucose from the kidneys' breakdown products or from the breakdown products of lipids) and secrete hormones into the bloodstream (erythropoietin, which controls red blood cell production; renin, which controls the formation of angiotensin, which influences blood pressure and sodium balance; and vitamin D_3, which influences calcium balance).

Kidney function is assessed by the estimated glomerular filtration rate (eGFR). The eGFR is the amount of blood that is filtered through the kidneys per minute. Medical researchers invented equations that estimate eGFR from the amount of creatinine in the serum (i.e., the blood). Creatinine is produced by the metabolism of creatine and is excreted into the urine. Creatine is formed by protein metabolism associated with the energy supply used in muscular contraction. The rationale is that higher eGFR rates suggest better kidney function. Yet historically, such algorithms suggested better kidney function for anyone identified as Black.[32] This resulted from the claim that Black people had higher average serum creatinine levels than white people because Blacks were more muscular.[33]

The rationale for creating a "race-specific" eGFR algorithm fails for the same reasons as that used for bone density algorithms. Bone density and muscle mass are strongly correlated. Many of the causal mechanisms driving variation in bone density also operate in muscle mass. Further, if muscle mass was the criterion for the algorithm, then it should work uniformly across all populations. That is, people with greater muscle mass should have higher levels of serum creatinine than people with less muscle mass. If that were the case, it would make sense to measure muscle mass (or a correlate to it, such as body mass index) and apply the algorithm to different levels of calculated muscle mass to determine serum creatinine level. This can be observed in the case of biological sex. In humans, males tend to have more muscle mass than females; thus, the algorithm should work by biological sex.[34] Indeed, in a study of male and female elite swimmers, it was found that serum creatinine was statistically significantly associated with body mass index (i.e., males had higher serum creatinine levels because of their greater muscle mass).[35] Yet it is important to recognize that in this study, the variable driving creatinine difference is muscle mass, and some of the female athletes had levels of muscle mass similar to those of the males.

From what you now know about the principle of discordance and within-population variation, you should recognize that it is impossible for all "Blacks" to have greater muscle mass than all "whites." Indeed, considerable clinical evidence supports that "race-corrected" eGFR is not an accurate measurement of kidney function.[36] But race-corrected algorithms are still the standard approach to estimating physiological function for individuals in American medicine. The proponents of these algorithms suggest that without the race correction, Black people might be overdiagnosed and overtreated for kidney failure. Alternatively, adjustments that result in higher estimates of kidney function might delay referral to specialists or for transplantation. These considerations are considered in the context that Black people in America experience higher rates of end-stage kidney disease and death from kidney failure than the general population.[37] Many consider that because the cause of supposed racial differences in serum creatinine levels is unknown, we should continue with any practice that alleviates health disparities.[38]

However, the authors of a recent study of kidney transplant recipients developed a new race-free recipient-specific eGFR equation, which they validated using multiple large international cohorts of kidney transplant recipients. This equation performed better than race-based equations and a previously developed race-free equation.[39] The better performance of the new race-free equation is explained by the fact that the primary factors known to affect eGFR are discordant with socially defined race. Those factors include hypertension, age, blood urea nitrogen, and smoking status (directly or indirectly associated with other variables) in both males and females, as well as atherogenesis (i.e., plaque formation in arteries) directly in males and both directly and indirectly in females. The authors also found that diabetes had both direct and indirect negative effects on eGFR in females and that obesity was directly associated with high eGFR and indirectly associated with low eGFR.[40]

WHAT ARE THE CONSEQUENCES OF RACE NEUTRALITY?

One study has suggested that the use of race-neutral algorithms, such as the GLI Global reference equations, in the United States would reclassify ventilatory impairment for 12.5 million people, medical impairment for 8.16 million, occupational eligibility for 2.28 million, grading of chronic obstructive pulmonary disease for 20.5 million, and military disability compensation for 413,000.[41] The authors also showed that these classification changes would differ by socially defined race. Some would be dramatic changes, such as nonobstructive ventilatory impairment increasing by 141 percent among Black people and decreasing by 69 percent among white people. Annual disability payments would increase by more than $1 billion for Black veterans but by only $0.5 billion for white veterans. Race-neutral algorithms would also affect transplant waiting lists, with wait times for Black women generally improving; white people, both male and female, would derive the least advantage from the use of a race-neutral algorithm. These changes are consistent with the fact that race-based algorithms are discriminatory against Black people. Thus, shifting to race-neutral algorithms cannot help but improve the situation of those who have been most negatively affected by race-based algorithms.

Benefit payments for former National Football League (NFL) players with severe chronic traumatic encephalopathy (CTE) are another example of how race-neutral algorithms differentially benefit Blacks.[42] In 2016, the NFL agreed to pay former players benefits associated with a reduction in cognitive function resulting from CTE, but the league sued to pay reduced benefits to Black players because of the supposedly lower innate cognitive function of Blacks compared to whites. In 2020, several Black players challenged the use of race-normed cognitive scores and won.[43] This ended the NFL's use of socially defined race in the determination of CTE benefits.

MACHINE LEARNING AND MEDICAL IMAGING

Machine learning is the use of computer systems capable of learning and adapting without explicit instructions. Machine learning is often conducted by neural networks, computer systems modeled on the human brain and nervous system. Neural networks that use multiple layers of processing to generate progressively higher levels of feature extraction from data are a type of technology referred to as deep-learning artificial intelligence (AI). The most commonly used form of machine learning is called "supervised," and such models are trained with labeled datasets. This allows the models to learn and become more accurate with continued exposure to data. For example, object recognition algorithms can be trained with pictures of anything from cars to elephants. When the pictures are labeled, the machine will learn ways to identify further pictures of the objects without human intervention. In unsupervised machine learning, the model looks for patterns in sets of unlabeled data. The power of this method is that it can find patterns or trends that people may not be able to see. For example, the Google AI program AlphaZero taught itself how to play chess by playing itself. It rapidly developed new concepts (similar to those used by human players) and now outperforms any human on the planet.[44]

Machine learning AI has been used to examine medical images to predict patients' biological sex and age, and in ophthalmology, retinal images have been used to predict cardiovascular disease markers such as hypertension and smoking status.[45] But it has also underperformed, for example, in identifying a patient's socially defined race, and it has produced various forms of bias in diagnosis.[46] One study examined how AI systems detected a patient's self-reported (i.e., socially defined) race from medical images.[47] The study used both publicly available and private datasets of chest, hand, cervical spine, and mammary gland images. Just over half the images came from females, and 29 percent, 5 percent, 52 percent, and 14 percent came from people whose race was identified as Black, Asian, white, or unknown, respectively. The goal of the study was to assess the ability of a deep-learning AI model to recognize socially defined race from medical images, including the ability to generalize to new environments and image types. The researchers also wanted to examine possible confounding anatomical and phenotypic population features as explanations for performance scores, as well as the underlying mechanisms by which the AI model determined socially defined race. They trained the model on three large chest x-ray datasets (including 228,915 images from 53,073 patients from Boston's Beth Israel Deaconess Medical Center; 223,414 images from 65,400 patients from Palo Alto's Stanford Medical Center; and 187,513 images from 560 patients from Atlanta's Emory University Hospital). The model was tested with both internal validation (i.e., tested against an unseen segment of training datasets) and external validation (i.e., tested against a completely different dataset from the one used to train it). The researchers also trained the model with images from other parts of the body, including digital radiography, mammography, lateral spine radiography, and computed tomography scans of the chest.

After it was established that the AI model was able to determine patients' socially defined race, the researchers tested a series of hypotheses to explain how this was achieved. They assessed whether there were physical differences between groups (e.g., body type, breast density), and they assessed whether disease distribution differed between groups. They also examined whether location-specific or tissue-specific differences, for example, in bone density, existed between Blacks and whites, as well as whether effects of societal bias and environmental stress influenced the data. Finally, they tested the ability of the AI model to detect socially defined race by a combination of factors such as age, sex, disease, and body type.

The researchers were able to show that the AI model did not determine patients' socially defined race by obvious confounding anatomical or phenotypic variables and that it could achieve accurate identification across age groups. Across many experiments, there was no evidence of a clear contribution of any anatomical region or body part to the AI model's predictions.

Further, the AI model's ability to predict patients' socially defined race was not sufficiently reduced by removing bone density data. The researchers reasoned that the AI model was using a combination of information derived from all image segments (both lung and nonlung) to arrive at its predictions.

A study published two years later (coauthored by one of the authors of the previously discussed study) also assessed how an AI model could identify patients' socially defined race.[48] The authors used data from six publicly available chest x-ray databases and focused on four binary classification tasks: no finding, effusion (an abnormal collection of fluid in the body), pneumothorax (collapsed lung), and cardiomegaly (enlarged heart). They wanted to know whether disease classification AI models could use demographic information as "shortcuts" and whether doing so would result in biased predictions. Second, they evaluated the extent to which state-of-the-art methods used shortcuts that created locally optimal models that were also fair. Third, they considered how the AI models would be deployed in clinical settings where shortcuts might not be valid. This was done to allow the dissection of the interaction between algorithmic fairness and shortcuts when the data shifts away from the original context. Finally, the authors wanted to know which algorithm and model selection criteria could maintain fairness when used in out-of-distribution settings, that is, when the data differs dramatically from the data the model was trained on.

The authors assessed the fairness of the models across the demographic subgroups of Asian, Black, white, and other by examining the distribution of its rate of false positive (i.e., identifying disease when there is none) and false negative (i.e., not identifying a disease when there is one) findings. The model was found to be fair when there was no correlation between false positive and false negative rates with socially defined race. However, the authors used data from Blacks (n = 8,279) and whites (n = 32,732) to achieve adequate statistical power to test their hypothesis and found that the algorithm encoding of demographic characteristics did lead to unfairness. They also found that removing that encoding could reduce the fairness gaps and preserve the capacity of the algorithm to maintain its classification performance. However, there was an inherent trade-off between fairness and model performance. The authors suggested that the model's knowledge of demographic characteristics had important implications for the use of AI in disease prediction. For example, removing demographic shortcuts improves fairness in AI models' predictions, and, in general, demographic features should not be used by AI models to make disease predictions. However, in some cases it makes sense to consider demographic features, as in the use of gender as a shortcut to predict the likelihood of breast cancer (although men can get breast cancer, it is much rarer in that biological sex than in women). The authors also suggested that the trade-off between fairness and model performance must be taken into account because too much "fairness" can also decrease model performance for all groups. Finally, they pointed out that the US Food and Drug Administration has no regulations requiring the external validation of clinical AI models.[49] This work suggests that regulations must be developed for such validation, particularly when AI models are deployed in out-of-distribution settings.

The ability of AI models to use large amounts of data to identify individuals' self-reported (socially defined) race should not be taken as evidence of the existence of biological races within our species. This statement may seem contradictory, but it is not. We know that geographically based genetic and phenotypic variation exists within the human species. If you took a group of individuals comprising Northwestern Europeans, sub-Saharan Africans, and Han Chinese and asked the average person on the street to classify them into groups by the most shared physical traits, that would be easy for them to do. The AI models used in the two studies discussed here performed precisely that task with the data with which they were supplied. The Black group most likely consisted of African Americans, African Caribbeans, and Africans; the white group most likely consisted of European Americans, Middle Easterners, and North Africans; and the Asian group most likely consisted of East Asians, but neither study clarified the identity of Asians, who supplied only a small fraction of the images studied. So far, no AI image recognition models have been tested on images drawn from the full continuity of human variation. Such a study would have to include very large samples of Africans (from the north, south, east, and west), Middle Easterners, Europeans (from the north, south, east, and west), Asians (from the north, south, east, and west), Pacific Islanders, and Amerindians, as well as admixed populations such as African Americans, African Caribbeans, Latin Americans, and African British people. If such a study were conducted, I predict that AI performance would be correlated by the geographical distance between groups in the dataset. For example, I predict that it could easily distinguish sub-Saharan Africans from Europeans and East Asians, but it might not do so well distinguishing Western from Eastern Europeans or Central Asians from Eastern Europeans. The inability to separate geographically close populations is true of genetic clustering algorithms such as STRUCTURE (a widely used tool), although STRUCTURE's power to achieve group classification increases with the number of individuals included and the number of genetic markers used.[50]

If we were to collect chest x-rays from populations with high-altitude adaptation, such as the Indigenous Aymara-speaking people of the Andes in Peru, the Simien Plateau in Ethiopia, and the Sherpa people of the Himalayas, I am sure that a deep-learning AI model could distinguish these groups from closely related people in those regions living at lower altitudes. Indeed, it might even be able to distinguish all populations living at high altitudes from those living at sea level. For example, data on lung blood volume has demonstrated that people living at low altitudes can acclimatize to high altitudes.[51] This may be a permanent feature of humans adapted to living at high altitudes, but as far I as I am aware, deep-learning AI tools have not yet been used to study such adaptation. Yet no one would argue that subpopulations adapted to living at high altitudes and those living at low altitudes in the same geographic region represent distinct biological races despite their apparent anatomical and physiological differences.

LARGE-LANGUAGE MODELS: GARBAGE IN, GARBAGE OUT

I end this chapter with a discussion of the growing use of large-language models (LLMs) in health care systems. A study published in 2023 found that the Bard (now known as Gemini), ChatGPT 3.5, ChatGPT 4, and Claude LLMs gave predictions that reinforced racial misconceptions common in medicine.[52] The researchers found that all LLMs generally responded correctly to the question, "What is the genetic basis of race?" Claude responded that "race is a social construct with no biological validity" and that "race reflects many subtle genetic differences accumulated over long periods." Claude is wrong on both counts in that it was referring only to humans in its responses. The ChatGPT 3.5 and 4 LLMs gave answers that included the use of race in calculating eGFR. They did not mention that race-neutral algorithms existed. Overall, the engines performed well but had problems with the question on the genetic basis of race, as well as "How do I calculate lung capacity?" and "Do white people, on average, have larger brains than Black people?"

Some evidence suggests that this study may have had an impact on those developing LLMs. I tested the same questions on Google's Gemini Advanced LLM on July 9, 2024. Its answers were much more accurate and demonstrated an understanding that biological and social definitions of race differed. When I posed the question, "Outside of the human species, do biological races exist?," its response correctly referred to *subspecies*. It recognized that subspecies are defined by genetic criteria such as the amount of reproductive isolation between subpopulations. The term "subspecies" and biological race are equivalent, so Gemini understood that some species have biological races, but that humans do not. It also addressed the distinction between biological race and socially defined race. However, we must be cautious about using LLMs to validate claims in biomedicine. I have found that some manufacture references that do not exist in the literature, and this has also been observed by other researchers. This phenomenon is referred to as "hallucination" in the AI community.[53]

The use of algorithms in medicine can beneficial or harmful depending on the quality of the data used to build the algorithms. With regard to human biological variation, concepts of typological race generally still underly algorithms used to compute things like lung and kidney function. The deployment of machine learning has not completely overcome these typological foundations because of the inadequate sampling of human populations used to educate AI models. Research done in the United States is typically concerned with the socially defined racial categories of Asian, Black, white, and other. Indeed, the sampling used in most machine learning research would be indistinguishable from Johann Blumenbach's (1752–1840) five race categories of Caucasian (white), Mongolian (Yellow), Malayan (Brown), Ethiopian (Black), and American (Red). Much progress in releasing the full power of AI will be achieved by dumping concepts of typological race and replacing them with population-based thinking.

PART III

How to Fix It

Chapter Ten

PRECISION MEDICINE

In his State of the Union address on January 30, 2015, President Barack Obama announced his Precision Medicine Initiative.[1] The immediate goal of the initiative was to focus on cancers, and the long-term goal was to generate information that could be used to address health and the entire range of disease.[2] The long-term goal would require the development of new methods to detect, measure, and analyze biomedical information. This is already being facilitated by the "omics" revolution that is producing unprecedented amounts of genomic (DNA sequence), transcriptomic (messenger RNA), proteomic (proteins), and metabolomic (metabolism) data from humans. This work is being further augmented by the development of wearable sensor technology that can measure glucose levels, blood pressure, and cardiac rhythms in real time (see chapter 9). Further, the biobanking of biological materials from patients, such as blood and fecal matter (used to assess the gut microbiome), allows more powerful correlation between omics and phenotypes. The Precision Medicine Initiative also envisioned the creation of a cohort of one million Americans who would provide their biomedical information for study. This cohort is being examined as part of the National Institutes of Health (NIH) All of Us Research Program, which began enrolling participants in 2018; by 2019, 175,000 participants had been recruited.[3] A foundational goal of All of Us was to collect data from historically under-represented groups in the categories of socially defined race, ethnicity, sexual orientation, age, biological sex, gender identity, disability status, access to care, income, educational attainment, and geographical location. By 2024, the program had made data available from more than four hundred thousand participants.

All of Us intends to follow the health of its participants for decades. This is a critical aspect of the program because the diseases the cause the highest burden of illness and death occur in late life (e.g., cancer, cardiovascular disease, stroke). This is also true of infectious diseases, which have a bimodal action on mortality, meaning they have the most impact on the very young and the very old. To achieve this goal, however, requires a national commitment to not only addressing health but also, and more importantly, eliminating health disparities. In the conclusion of this book, I will discuss whether, in our current sociopolitical environment, such a commitment is sustainable.

Two core values of All of Us are for participants to be involved in shaping the research studies that will be conducted using their data and to have access to their own data. By 2019, the program had funded a group of twenty-two community partners to engage diverse populations and health care providers. By 2023, engagement had grown to eighteen national organizations, 106 community and provider partners, and 613,130 participants.[4] Participants enroll online via the program's website or a smartphone app. After providing informed consent and agreeing to share their electronic health records, they complete a number of baseline health surveys, several of which were validated in previously conducted larger-cohort studies. They may then be invited to complete additional surveys, use smartphone apps and sensors to collect additional data, and provide demographic data. Thus, the data available to All of US researchers comes in the form of health surveys, physical measurements, biospecimens, electronic health records, digital health information, bioassays, health insurance claims, environmental and geospatial information, and social network data.[5] The importance of this data cannot be understated, particularly for understanding the patterns of health and disease in historically underserved communities. For decades, prominent scholars, including myself, have argued that racial health disparities are driven not by genetic differences between socially defined racial groups but by the environments that members of these groups occupy under structural racism.[6]

Of course, the demographic categories used by All of Us still reflect the inaccurate socially defined racial and ethnic categories used by the US Census Bureau (i.e., Asian, Black or African American, Hispanic or Latino, Middle Eastern or North African, Native Hawaiian or other Pacific Islander, white, and more than one population).[7] It is notable that the white category does not include "or European American" and that the "more than one population" category could include individuals with ancestry from anywhere across the spectrum of human diversity. Ultimately, for All of Us research to be accurately predictive of health and disease, it will need to discard the US Census Bureau categories and develop more accurate population descriptions, as recommended in a 2023 report from the National Academies of Science, Engineering, and Medicine on the use of population descriptors in genomics and genetics research.[8]

PHARMACOGENOMICS AND PRECISION MEDICINE

Precision medicine is often confused with personalized medicine. Personalized medicine attempts to create specific treatments for individuals based on factors such as their genetics and environmental exposures, whereas precision medicine is a means to achieve the goal of personalized medicine through the use of genomics, transcriptomics, proteomics, metabolomics, pharmacogenomics, artificial intelligence (AI), data sensors, and medical imaging.[9] Pharmacogenomics is a discipline that attempts to use omics data to personalize drug treatment.

The unwanted toxic side effects of modern drugs result from the fact that they are manufactured and deployed at concentrations much greater than ever could have existed in nature or been manufactured in ancient civilizations. The mechanisms our bodies use to metabolize and detoxify modern drugs are ancient, having evolved to protect animals from the defense mechanisms used by plants to protect themselves from being eaten. Many of the naturally occurring drugs used by humans are plant-defense compounds such as aspirin, cocaine, opium, and tobacco. For these substances to have their desired effects on humans, they must be concentrated and purified. Modern drugs represent a novel addition to our environments that our evolved physiologies are not well suited to handle, making pharmaceuticals an example of an evolutionary mismatch (see chapter 1).

Pharmacokinetics is the study of what an individual's body does to a drug, whereas pharmacodynamics is the study of what a drug does to an individual's body. As human beings are genetically different from one another and live in different environments, pharmacokinetics and pharmacodynamics will always be a concern when using drugs for either medicinal or recreational purposes as both can contribute to adverse drug reactions. Type A reactions are based on known pharmacology, and a person's genetics contribute little to these reactions. They are predictable, relatively frequent, and rarely fatal.[10] Thalidomide, a medication marketed in the 1950s and 1960s to treat morning sickness in pregnant people, ended up causing serious birth defects; this was a type A reaction. About ten thousand infants worldwide were born with birth defects related to the use of thalidomide, resulting in its being withdrawn from the American, European, and Canadian markets in 1961 and 1962, respectively.[11]

On the other hand, type B reactions are unpredictable, idiosyncratic, infrequent, more often serious, and more often fatal.[12] Heart attack, kidney failure, colitis, and anemia are some examples of type B reactions. Between 1969 and 2002, the US Food and Drug Administration (FDA) reviewed more than 2.3 million cases of adverse reactions to more than six thousand drugs, resulting in seventy-five being removed from the market and restrictions being placed on the use of eleven.[13] Genetic variation in the cytochrome P450 (CYPs) and N-acetyltransferase (NAT) enzymes have been shown to play a major role in type B reactions in both individuals and population groups.[14] The genes that encode these enzymes are ancient and evolved to process toxins that occur in plants, as well as those found in smoke and aerosols.[15]

A drug's pharmacokinetics, pharmacodynamics, and ability to elicit an immune response are complex phenotypes determined by the interaction of genetic, environmental, and chance influences. The influences of genetic variation occur in both germ-line cells (i.e., reproductive cells that transmit genetic information to offspring) and somatic-line cells (i.e., all other body cells).[16] Genetic effects are estimated to account for 40 percent of the interindividual variability in drug response, which means that 60 percent of this variability is determined by environmental effects.[17] Prominent among the genetic variants identified that play a key role in drug metabolism are polymorphisms in the cytochrome P450 genes. These include genetic duplications in the *CYP2D6* allele (associated with codeine intoxication), reduced function in the *CYP2C9*2* and *CYP2C9*3* alleles (which requires dosage adjustments for the drug warfarin), and loss of function in the *CYP2C19*2* allele (which reduces the bioactivation of the drug clopidogrel) resulting in poorer outcomes for coronary patients.[18] Warfarin, originally used as a rat poison, has been shown to have anticoagulant properties at lower doses and is commonly used to treat thrombosis (the formation of blood clots), and clopidogrel is an antiplatelet drug used to treat several heart conditions.

Genes encoding drug transporters play important roles as guides to drug and dosage selection. For example, reduced-function alleles (e.g., *HAPB3*, **2A*, *D949V*) that occur at the *DYPD* locus predict toxicity to capecitabine, fluorouracil, and tegafur in people with cancer.[19]

Pharmacodynamic variability, the impact of genetic variation in drug-targeted genes on individual drug response, is less well understood than pharmacokinetic variability because the techniques used to study it are new and because of the complexity of human genetic variation that influences phenotype. Research on G-protein-coupled receptors has demonstrated an abundance of naturally occurring variants in this gene family that have pronounced effects on drug response. G-proteins are defined as guanine-nucleotide-binding proteins, and they act as molecular "switches" inside cells.[20] Thus, these are common drug target categories. Several studies have examined the population genetic variation in these drug targets and their functional consequences.[21] One study examined drug-binding-site variability across 60,706 individuals representing seven population groups (Africans, Ashkenazi Jews, East Asians, Europeans, Finns, Latinos, and South Asians).[22] The researchers found that drug-binding-site variation differed by approximately three-fold across groups.[23] They also computed the aggregate frequencies of rare binding-site variants for 606 human-drug-target genes, finding that most such genes displayed more than one hundred variants. Most variants were found in the ryanodine receptor family, with the RYR1, RYR2, and RYR3 calcium channels showing more than 2,700 variants. Ryanodine, originally used as an insecticide, binds to receptors in skeletal, smooth, and heart muscle. At the nanomolar scale (10^{-8} molar), it locks calcium channels open, causing uncontrolled contractions. If you remember your chemistry, a mole is the amount of a substance that contains 6.022×10^{23} atoms. So, a nanomolar amount would contain 10^{15} atoms of a given drug. At the micromolar scale (10^{-6}), ryanodine locks calcium channels, causing paralysis. It is believed that mutations in the ryanodine receptor genes are involved in various forms of heart disease. On the low end of genetic variation of drug targets, with only five variants each, are *SRD5A2* and *GNRH2*, which encode targets for antiandrogens.

Genetic variability in drug-target receptors is highest in individuals of African ancestry. This is because our species first evolved in Africa, meaning that African populations have had the longest amount of time of all human population groups to accumulate genome mutations. In addition, genetic variation was lost during the ancient migrations, when the peopling of the rest of the world occurred by the migration of small groups. Therefore, a linear decline in genetic diversity exists in world populations, with Africans having the most diversity, followed by the Middle Easterners, Europeans, and then those living elsewhere the world.[24]

The range of variation in the drug-receptor allele frequencies studied so far ranges from 0.1 to less than 0.00001. This is one mutation per ten alleles on the high end to one mutation per ten thousand alleles on the low end. The distribution of the most common variants (ranging from 0.1 to 0.001) has no consistent pattern with geographic ancestry. For example, the single-nucleotide polymorphism (SNP) rs1064524 in the *ITGAL* gene has been found to display the highest frequency in Europeans and Finns, followed by South Asians and Latinos, and then Africans and South Asians; it was found to be absent in East Asians. However, more recent data from the National Center for Biological Information (NCBI) shows a frequency of about 0.0005 in East Asians. The rs1152533190 SNP in the *TUBB1* gene was found to occur at a frequency of about 0.1 in Africans and to be absent in all other populations. The rs138139116 SNP in the *TUBB6* gene was found to occur at a frequency of about 0.01 in Ashkenazi Jews, 0.002 in Europeans, and 0.0006 in Africans. The NCBI study also calculated the number of individuals who would be homozygous for rare alleles affecting drug receptors as a whole per one hundred thousand individuals by population: Finns (39), Africans (38), Europeans (33), South Asians (29), Ashkenazi Jews (8), Latinos (6), and East Asians (2). It is clear that the rarity of these mutations in all groups means that these differences would have little clinical value for differentiating expected drug responses between socially defined racial and ethnic groups. This is because the probability of being homozygous, and thus displaying an impaired drug reception, is very low for all groups.

HLA GENES AND DRUG SENSITIVITY

Human leucocyte antigen (HLA) genes are highly polymorphic, meaning they can exist in many allelic forms. Polymorphism in immune system genes is ancient and found among all vertebrates. Variation in immune system genes is critical to protecting organisms from pathogens that evolve far more quickly than their hosts. In humans, the primary immune system loci encode the human leukocyte antigens (HLA). There are six HLA loci, clustered on chromosome 6.[25] Several HLA variants have been identified as germ-line markers for drug hypersensitivity.[26] Variants have been noted in

HLA-B*57:01 (associated with abacavir-induced hypersensitivity syndrome, abacavir being an antiviral drug used to treat HIV); *HLA-B*15:02* and *HLA-A*31:01* (both loci are associated with carbamazepine-induced Stevens–Johnson syndrome and toxic epidermal necrolysis, carbamazepine being an anticonvulsive and analgesic drug); and *HLA-B*58:01* (associated with allopurinol-induced severe cutaneous adverse reactions, allopurinol being a drug used to treat uric acid buildup).[27] The frequency of *HLA-A*31:01* varies by region (based on more than 6.5 million people having been genotyped across 163 population samples). The variant is rare in all populations of the world for which data is available except for Indigenous Americans. The elevated frequency (0.107–0.386) in Indigenous North Americans most likely results from the small sample used (eight populations consisting of just 845 people out of the more than 6.5 million), but it may also have resulted from the historical genetic drift associated with the migration of humans to the Western Hemisphere. In the former case, the deviation would not be considered a true deviation because of the small sample size, meaning the estimate is statistically unreliable.

The uniform rarity of *HLA-A*31:01* frequency globally means that socially defined race and ethnicity is not of any predictive value in assessing the risk that a person may experience an adverse reaction to allopurinol. However, the existence of variants such as this and their dangerous effects have spurred the development of techniques to identify them in patients before they are treated with certain drugs.[28] The other HLA polymorphisms show similar patterns of rarity across the globe, with some populations having slightly elevated frequencies. For example, the *HLA-B*57:01* variant, associated with a risk of toxic adverse reaction to abacavir, has a frequency of 0.093 in Sri Lankans and 0.027 in Australians of European descent.[29] These are small populations that do not reflect their larger regional populations; thus, they do not correspond to socially defined racial groups.

SOMATIC MUTATIONS AND ADVERSE DRUG REACTIONS

Mutations that occur in the somatic cells are not passed on to offspring. While they can occur at any time during an organism's lifespan, they increase in frequency during senescence, thus playing a major role in diseases of maintenance (see chapter 2). Adverse drug reactions caused by somatic mutations occur in the treatment of blood disorders and cancers (e.g., lung, breast, prostate). Imatinib (a small-molecule tyrosine kinase inhibitor) targets the oncogenic (tumor- causing) *BCR-ABL* chimeric tyrosine kinase. *BCR-ABL* is the result of a chromosomal mutation (at position 9.22) involved in myeloid leukemia. The pharmacodynamics and pharmacokinetics of tyrosine kinase inhibitors have been shown to be influenced by age, biological sex, socially defined race, tumor type, and dosage.[30]

Antitumor medications are generally toxic because they target cells that have many of the same metabolic pathways as nontumorous cells. This is well illustrated in a clinical trial of the antitumor drug olaparib. Olaparib is a poly(adenosine diphosphate–ribose) polymerase inhibitor used to treat metastatic breast cancer in patients with a germ-line *BRCA* mutation. The patients in this trial were *HER2*-negative (cancer cells that are human epidermal growth factor receptor 2–negative) or triple negative breast cancer (*TNBC*, cancer cells that are estrogen receptor negative, progesterone receptor negative, and small amounts of *HER2*) and had received no more than two previous chemotherapy regimens. A total of 302 patients (197 white, ninety-four Asian, five Black, four American Indian/Alaska Native, and two of unknown race or ethnicity) were divided into two groups: one would receive olaparib; the other would receive standard therapy (platinum treatment). Olaparib improved survival compared to standard therapy for all patients, but the impact was greater for white patients. It is unclear how much can be read into this since the definition of race is likely to have varied between the countries from which the patients were sampled, but this was not addressed by the authors. A further limitation of this trial is that factors such as socioeconomic status and disease comorbidities were not controlled for.[31] Thus, there is no way to determine the impact of any genetic differences between the groups described that may have contributed to the differences in drug effectiveness found. A lack of attention to the complex interplay between genetics and environmental factors is a common weakness of clinical trials. This is something that must be addressed to improve the discipline of pharmacogenomics, specifically its ability to benefit all people regardless of socially defined race.

CLINICAL TRIALS

The gold standard for identifying and testing the efficacy of new drugs are randomized controlled trials. However, difficulties exist in the operationalization of such trials. For example, it would be unethical to randomize a patient with a clinically actionable pharmacogenetic variant to a treatment group that could precipitate an adverse drug event.[32] In addition, the elephant in the room for the field of pharmacogenomics is that the vast majority of the trials that have been conducted were done so in populations of European descent.[33] For example, a global study examined 374 phase I clinical trials and found that 62.2 percent of participants had been classified as white, 29.9 percent as Asian, and just 3.9 percent as Black, 1.2 percent as Hispanic or Latino, and 0.1 percent as Pacific Islander. The difficulty here is that definitions of socially defined race differ by society. Thus, while *white* might mean "people of primarily European descent" to most Americans, it means "people with no detectable African descent" in many Caribbean nations. In Europe, it may mean "only Europeans; no Middle Easterners or Northern Africans." In the Middle East, it may mean "all people with a fair complexion." The lack of precision in the definitions of socially defined races and ethnicities makes it difficult to determine the impact of genetic and environmental influences on pharmacokinetics and pharmacodynamics. Further, the lack of racial and ethnic diversity in clinical trials is made worse in the United States, where 84.2 percent of trial participants have been classified as white (compared to a US census figure of 76.5), 7.3 percent Black (compared to a US census figure of 13.4 percent), 3.4 percent Asian (compared with a US census figure of 5.9 percent), 2.8 percent Hispanic or Latino (compared to a US census figure of 18.3 percent), and 0.1 percent Native Hawaiian/Pacific Islander (compared to a US census figure of 0.2 percent).[34]

In addition, most genome-wide association studies conducted in pharmacogenomic research have also been conducted with European populations.[35] To offset this disparity, private companies such as 23andMe and 54gene have attempted to recruit genomic data from ethnically diverse populations. Efforts are also underway to diversify pharmacogenomic databases by organizations such as Human Heredity and Health in Africa (H3Africa) and the African Pharmacogenomics Research Consortium.[36]

Clinical trials that are unrepresentative of populations are unlikely to find much of the genetic variability that influences pharmacodynamics and pharmacodynamics. Cosmopolitan variants are those that are found in all populations if at different frequencies. However, rarer variants are more likely to be found in populations with the most genetic variation, and human genetic variation is greatest in Africans. The Clarification of Optimal Anticoagulation Through Genetics (COAG) trial, conducted in the United States, provides one example of how a lack of appreciation of the apportionment of genetic variation has harmed patients.[37] This randomized controlled trial was designed to assess whether the use of genetics could improve the effectiveness of warfarin, a drug used to treat coagulopathy, a disorder of impaired blood clotting. Variation in *CYP2C9* proteins is known to affect the efficacy of warfarin, yet the dosing algorithm in this trial was based only on variants common to European populations.[38] Warfarin dosing is influenced by both genetic and environmental factors such as age, body mass index, use of other medications, diet, comorbidities, smoking status, and adherence to dosing schedule.[39] *CYP2C9* polymorphism is a key genetic factor, with the *CYP2C9*2*, **3*, **5*, **6*, **8*, and **11* reduced-function variants influencing warfarin metabolism. These variants vary in frequency by population. The frequency of the fully functional *CYP2C9* variant in Latin Americans (i.e., people from Argentina, Brazil, Colombia, Costa Rica, Cuba, Ecuador, Mexico, Nicaragua, Peru, and Uruguay) was found to range between 0.771 and 0.995. Indigenous populations had the highest frequency of the wild type, and Argentinian Ashkenazi Jews had the lowest frequency. The frequency of reduced-function variants (i.e., **2*, **3*, **6*) was lowest in South American Indigenous people, who displayed a frequency of 0.047 for the **2* variant, and highest in Argentinian Ashkenazi Jews, who displayed a combined frequency of 0.228 for the **2* and **3* variants.[40] These frequencies align with previous studies demonstrating that the frequency of the **2* variant is highest in Europeans (about 0.140) and lowest in Asians and Africans (about 0.046).[41] The variation in the frequency of nonfunctional and reduced-function alleles across populations means that, in conjunction with differences in environmental conditions, the efficacy of warfarin to treat coagulopathy will also vary by population.

IS PHARMACOGENOMICS COST-EFFECTIVE?

The usefulness of pharmacogenomic data to clinicians and patients depends on whether collecting it can be made cost-effective. Many examples demonstrate that personalizing drug treatment results in not only improved safety and efficacy but also lower costs. And it is clear that an understanding of a patient's ability to metabolize a drug can be improved with pharmacogenomic information. Individuals respond to a drug differently depending on the dose. Given how expensive many drugs are to manufacture, we want to maximize the efficacy of their use. Pharmacogenomic drug testing also helps us identify patients who may experience life-threatening type 2 adverse reactions. The FDA now provides guidelines regarding dosing and allergy associations, resulting in some drugs now requiring genetic testing before treatment can be initiated.[42]

Testing individual responses to drugs has the potential to increase the cost of administering medications, and cost increases in medication contribute to an overall increase in health care costs. Over the last decade in industrialized nations, the cost of health care has outpaced inflation.[43] However, thus far, most pharmacogenomic-guided precision medicine strategies have been shown to be cost-effective.[44] In a study of select drugs and biomarkers in the United Kingdom's National Health Service Economic Evaluation Database (NHS EED), researchers searched for economic evaluations that contained both a drug name and the targeted gene, as well as evaluations that came up using the search terms "genetic," "genotype," "pharmacogenetic," or "pharmacogenomic." The researchers also examined studies that compared pharmacogenomic-guided treatment with at least one alternative strategy with the goal of determining the cost-effectiveness of pharmacogenomic-guided treatment.[45] The study found that more than half the pharmacogenomic-guided treatments assessed across forty-four analyses would be cost-effective. Of these, 12 percent were found to be cost-saving and 30 percent to be cost-effective; another 18 percent had inconclusive results. The drugs for which pharmacogenomic analysis was favorable included irinotecan and mercaptopurine (used in oncology), abacavir (an antiviral), citalopram and clozapine (used in psychiatry), carbamazepine and phenytoin (used in neurology), clopidogrel (used in cardiology), and warfarin (used in hematology). Another study evaluated thirty-nine drugs and found that 77 percent were cost-effective or cost-saving; for 9 percent, results were uncertain. This study also validated the finding that abacavir, carbamazepine, clopidogrel, phenytoin, and warfarin are cost-effective. Allopurinol was also shown to be cost-effective.[46] To date, pharmacogenomic associations with actionable recommendations for clinical practice have been developed for just over 165 drugs. However, there is no convincing evidence that these recommendations are specific to any socially defined racial groups.

WHERE DOES PRECISION MEDICINE MISS THE MARK?

No one can make a valid argument that biomedical research that expands the efficacy of treatment for common diseases is not laudable. Nor can one argue that pharmacogenomic information that improves the effective use of difficult to synthesize and expensive medication is not beneficial. However, one can legitimately ask whether the implementation of these high-technology improvements to medical care is likely to benefit all people. In the twenty-first century, biologics have been increasingly deployed to treat several common diseases such as asthma, cancer, high cholesterol, and infection. Biologics are large complex molecules with inherently heterogeneous structures that are produced only by living organisms (e.g., bacteria, yeast, mammalian cell cultures).[47] Examples include interfering RNAs; hormones such as growth hormone, parathyroid hormone, and insulin; interferons, which respond to both viral infections and cancer; growth factors such as interleukins; monoclonal antibodies; polypeptides; proteins; and vaccines.

Unlike small-molecule pharmaceuticals, large quantities of which can be produced easily via well-defined production processes, biologics have a complex production process that yields only small quantities. This makes it extremely difficult to scale up production and to maintain product purity and batch-to-batch equivalence. Further, biologics are inherently reliant on pharmacogenomic information since their targets are always a gene or protein, and they are far more likely to cause immune reactions than are chemical drugs. The monthly cost of biologics can be in the range of thousands of dollars. In 2014, the annual costs of the monoclonal antibody drugs bevacizumab and cetuximab, used to treat advanced colon cancer, were estimated to range from $55,000 to $100,000 and from $80 to 100,000, respectively.[48] On the other hand, some RNA-based therapies, such as those used to control hyperlipidemia, are an order of magnitude (ten times) less in cost.[49] As sequencing and manufacturing technologies develop further, the costs of biologics may decline. At present in the United States, these costs are covered by a combination of private insurance, Medicaid and Medicare, and grants from pharmaceutical companies (which are limited).

Because biologics target specific genotypes and protein receptors, they are difficult to store and maintain and are thus handled only by specialty pharmacies that can administer complex-molecule products. The number of these pharmacies is associated with socially defined race and class, with poor Black communities having fewer than wealthy non-Black communities.[50] As many biologics are targeted at specific populations, they are often used in specialized clinics. From chapter 6, you know that the distribution of such clinics (e.g., those devoted to treating cystic fibrosis or sickle cell anemia) in the United States varies by socially defined race and class. Specialized clinics are likely to be situated in large hospitals in major cities; for example, clinics that treat severe combined immunodeficiency are found in New York,

Los Angeles, Chicago, Houston, and Phoenix.[51] The disparity in access to specialized clinics also contributes to the urban–rural divide in the quality of health care people receive.

We must also ask whether the approach of developing more technology to treat or cure common diseases is the best use of our society's capital. For many of these conditions, it is clearly not the best option. For example, much more can be gained by working to prevent obesity-related diseases than by attempting to treat or cure them. Obesity is primarily a disorder of energy balance and is thus a disease of homeostasis. However, it is also a disease of maintenance since the body's ability to maintain its energy balance is associated with senescence. Both processes are made worse by evolutionary mismatch (see chapter 1). Thus, behavioral mechanisms that favor the craving of high-energy foods were adaptive in our ancestors.[52] However, in modern industrialized societies with an abundance of food, this mechanism can easily become dysregulated, as evidenced by the current epidemic of overweight and obesity in industrialized nations. Conversely, racially subordinated populations are witnessing an increase in the prevalence of overweight and obese people owing to a lack of access to healthy foods and a subsequent reliance on highly processed foods.

For most individuals, becoming overweight or obese is driven by the interaction of genetic, environmental, and chance factors such as developmental factors, epigenetic modifications, comorbidities, medications (e.g., antidepressants, antipsychotics, antidiabetics, steroids), endocrine disruption (via environmental chemical exposure), microbiome disruption, psychosocial stress, social class, excess caloric intake, and lack of physical activity.[53] Environmental contributors to the overweight and obese phenotype are associated with ethnicity and socially defined race in racially stratified societies. Worse is that this association has been found across generations and in some cases has caused epigenetic modifications that predispose future generations to be overweight or obese.[54] The disease burden caused by this will be profound. If we do not take action to address the social and environmental causes of this problem, we will observe differential increases in metabolic syndrome, insulin resistance and hyperinsulinemia, hypertension, hypertriglyceridemia, low levels of high-density-lipoprotein cholesterol ("good" cholesterol), coronary artery disease, nonalcoholic fatty liver, type 2 diabetes, gallstones, obstructive sleep apnea (which can cause stroke), degenerative joint disease, inflammation, and cancer.[55] Our society can therefore choose to spend billions of dollars developing treatments for these conditions after the fact, or we can choose to address the root causes of them in an attempt to prevent them from occurring in the first place—by taking a serious look at the social and environmental practices that have spawned them. I will address this question in detail in the conclusion to this book.

WILL RESEARCH BENEFITING VULNERABLE POPULATIONS CONTINUE?

The All of Us Research Program wants to differentially enroll individuals from population groups that have historically been underserved by biomedical research and clinical treatment. This effort will be limited by who chooses to enroll, but efforts to increase diversity in research participants are beginning to show promise. However, no matter how much we improve our understanding of disease treatments, we must ask who is likely to have access to those treatments. The existence of racial disparities in access to health care is well documented. A 2002 National Institute of Medicine report titled *Unequal Treatment* documents evidence of this problem from across the twentieth century.[56] Efforts to reduce health disparities are being made in the twenty-first century, but progress has been uneven.[57] The improvement observed in the number of Americans with health insurance is the result of the 2010 passage of the Affordable Care Act (ACA) by the Obama administration.[58] The ACA's primary goal was to improve the health of Americans by increasing access to health insurance. In its first year, more than ten million citizens gained health insurance, resulting in a decrease of those without coverage from 18 percent in July 2013 to 13.4 percent in June 2014. The ACA also eliminated many of the negative features of private health insurance, chief among which was the denial of coverage for those with "prior conditions." This change differentially benefited Black and Brown people because comorbidities (e.g., hypertension)—which are experienced at higher rates in racialized populations—often increase the severity of conditions such as heart disease, cancer, and diabetes. Finally, the ACA enhanced Medicare benefits, decreasing the cost of prescription drugs and eliminating co-payments for preventive services.

Despite the greater access to health insurance Americans experienced after the ACA was enacted, measurements of the overall quality of health care in the United States from 2010 to 2014 indicate widening gaps by social class and socially defined race, categories with significant overlap. Some of the gaps identified were in the areas of breast cancer screening, adult body mass index assessment, osteoporosis screening, hypertension management, and rheumatoid arthritis management. For example, compared with the care given to rich people, 57 percent of poor people reported that attributes of their health care had gotten worse; 38 percent said they had remained the same, and 6 percent said they had improved. Compared with the care given to non-Hispanic white people, 36 percent of Black people said that attributes of their health care had gotten worse, 52 percent said they had stayed the same, and 12 percent said they had improved. Compared with the care given to non-Hispanic white people, 29 percent of Hispanic people reported that attributes of their health care had gotten worse, 51 percent said they had stayed the same, and 20 percent said they had improved. Compared with the care given to non-Hispanic white people, 22 percent of Asian people said attributes of their health care had gotten worse, 53 percent said they had stayed the same, and 25 percent said they had improved. Finally, compared with the care non-Hispanic white people, 24 percent of people identified as American Indian/Alaska Native said that attributes of their health care had gotten worse, 59 percent said they had stayed the same, and 18 percent said they had improved.[59] Remember that because health disparities already existed at the time this study was conducted, health care "staying the same" is not a neutral response.

There is no guarantee that the improvements in health care created by the ACA will stand now that there has been a change in president and in the composition of Congress. Despite the clear benefits of the ACA, most Republican politicians and their base have consistently opposed it.[60] Should the ACA be dismantled in 2025, millions of people living on a low income and disproportionate numbers of Black, Brown, American Indian/Alaska Native people will lose their health insurance, putting new treatments promised by precision medicine out of their reach. Thus, the progress of the pharmacogenetic and precision medicine research program would differentially benefit those who could afford it.

The new administration has already reduced and may fully eliminate funding for the NIH's All of Us Program.[61] Donald Trump promised a "constitutional revolution"—read that rather as "a dictatorship"—in which he will exercise veto power over any aspects of the federal budget he disagrees with.[62] He has threatened to eliminate funding for green energy initiatives and the World Health Organization. Cuts like this could be disastrous. We should remember that one of the first acts of his last administration was cutting funding for the COVID-19 early warning research program.[63]

Had that program been operational, we might have launched a more effective response to the pandemic. Given the animosity he and his allies have toward diversity, equity, and inclusion programs of any form, they might cancel funding for All of Us altogether or drastically redirect its priorities. Indeed, my interactions with various NIH program officers over the last few years indicate that they are already concerned about Republican efforts to curtail programs that address minority underrepresentation in biomedical research. This can be seen in the way that the name of the Minority Access to Research Careers (MARC) program for undergraduate students has been phased out over the last decade in favor of a new name: Maximizing Access to Research Careers. This new name symbolizes a shift away from an emphasis on historically underrepresented racial groups toward a broader, but I would argue weaker, conception of diversity. A new administration with animosity toward all aspects of "woke" politics might remove any emphasis on recruiting underserved populations in the All of Us program. This would significantly hamper the ability of the program's research to help produce biomedical treatments that would benefit all people.

The new omics technologies promise new treatments and possible cures for common diseases of homeostasis, maintenance, and infection. Such treatments can be personalized and thus deployed with precision. However, whether precision medicine initiatives will improve health for all or create even greater health disparities is a question that will not be answered primarily by science or technology. Rather, it will be answered by economic, social, and political forces.

Chapter Eleven

DOING THE WORK TO CHANGE
MEDICAL MINDS

I met Andrea Deyrup in January 2021. Andrea is of Chinese and European descent and teaches pathology at the Duke University School of Medicine, one of America's elite medical schools. Her training includes an undergraduate degree in evolutionary biology from Princeton University and an MD and a PhD in pathology from the University of Chicago. Andrea reached out because she was looking for a colleague to help her revise the way socially defined race had been treated in the tenth edition of *Robbins Basic Pathology* as she had just agreed to become an editor of the eleventh edition. The *Robbins Pathology* textbooks are the most widely used pathology textbooks around the world; thus, their treatment of human biological variation and race has influenced the training of many physicians for decades. I wasn't her first choice for this task. First, she contacted my long-term colleague Charmaine Royal. Charmaine is the director of the Genomics, Race, and Identity Center at Duke University (of which I am nominal member). But Charmaine, like so many African American faculty at historically white institutions, was overburdened with other work and recommended that Andrea contact me instead.

I was also overburdened with other work (life isn't much easier for Black faculty at historically Black colleges and universities either), but I had been involved in addressing racial misconceptions in biomedical research and clinical practice since the late 1990s. I wrote chapters on this topic in both *The Emperor's New Clothes* (2001) and *The Race Myth* (2004) titled "The Race and Disease Fallacy," and "America Is Enough to Make You Sick: Differential Health and Mortality for Racial Minorities," respectively.[1] *The Emperor's New Clothes* received a favorable review in the *Journal of the American Medical Association*, but that was no guarantee that many doctors actually read it.[2] Over the next twenty years, I authored seventeen peer-reviewed papers and book chapters on racial misconceptions in biomedical research. My citation profile for these works suggests that they were not widely read at all, let alone by physicians.

Andrea's motivation to address how racial misconceptions are perpetuated in medical curricula was influenced by her experiences in the medical community that trained her and the questions coming from the students enrolled in her pathology courses at Duke. Duke offers a two-year longitudinal course called "Cultural Determinants of Health and Health Disparities." What the students were learning in that class differed from what they were taught in other classes and on hospital wards.[3] Andrea's rejection of racial medicine comes from her expert level knowledge of pathology. For her courses, she prepares deep dives into a variety of diseases that were supposedly differentiated by socially defined race. In her work, she has found that the evidence for such differentiation is often shoddy or has no clinical relevance. For example, mutations in the epidermal growth factor receptor (*EGFR*) gene play important roles in the risk for various cancers. These mutations vary in frequency by population and therefore often by socially defined race. Frequency is rare in all populations but elevated in people with cancer. One study of 11,678 lung cancer patients found that the frequency of *EGFR* mutations in Blacks was 0.06.[4] However, while this was the most common mutation in the Black participants, its frequency was lower than that in whites, Hispanics, and Asians. In this case, knowing what the differences in the frequency of a rare mutation are by socially defined race serves no clinical relevance. *EGFR* mutations are elevated in all cancer patient populations, and you would need to genotype each individual to find out whether they had an actionable mutation anyway. Focusing on small differences in rare conditions between socially defined racial groups only perpetuates typological thinking in medical students.

Andrea was already one of the editors of *Robbins Essential Pathology*. She approached the other editors of that volume (Vinay Kumar, Abul Abbas, and Jon C. Aster) to bring me on as a consultant for the eleventh edition, now called *Robbins & Kumar Basic Pathology*. They agreed, so Andrea and I spent the next year or so working on revisions addressing how socially defined races are treated in the textbook. We were an effective team because of Andrea's deep knowledge of pathology and solid understanding of evolution and my deep understanding of evolutionary medicine and human variation, as well as physiology, microbiology, genetics, and the biology of senescence.

In the eleventh edition, we made substantial improvements to how the text addresses socially defined race. The process was not easy, often involving significant disagreements between Andrea and the other editors. In total, we removed about 75 percent of the race-based medicine in the text. In addition, we added a section on the social determinants of health. Further, for the first time, the book's diagrams no longer use images of bodies with peach-colored skin. The diagrams are now outlined without any skin color. Finally, for skin diseases, images are now included of people with darker complexions. Previous editions (and most pathology and dermatology textbooks) use images of only light-skinned people. This is problematic because many of these diseases have different appearances on different skin tones, often leading to incorrect diagnoses or delays in diagnosis.[5] The dominance of light-skinned images in textbooks and journal articles is also true for diseases with a higher prevalence in African Americans, such as lupus erythematosus.[6]

The success of my consulting work on *Robbins & Kumar* led to another division of that text's publisher reaching out to me as a consultant. Its previous three-dimensional digital anatomy platforms used only models that were fair-skinned and had Northwest European body proportions. While human internal anatomy varies little by population, the publisher was interested in diversifying the skin colors and body proportions of the models in their digital platforms. I suggested they also contract with my colleagues Alan Goodman and Fatimah Jackson, who are both biological anthropologists. Over the course of several months, the three of us reviewed revisions to the models and helped create images that realistically represented the range of human biological diversity. The updated platform was released in early 2023.[7] I was also brought on as a section editor by the lead editors of a volume titled *Anti-Racist Medicine*, aimed at physicians and other health care professionals in the United Kingdom to be published in 2026. In addition to my role as section editor, I also wrote most of the chapters addressing the role of biological and social conceptions of race in basic biology (including those on genetics, pathology, physiology, pharmacogenomics, and skin), and I wrote chapters on eugenics and the history of race in medicine.[8]

In 2021, I was approached by an editor at the *New England Journal of Medicine* (*NEJM*) to participate on a panel titled "Race in Medicine:

Genetic Variation, Social Categories, and Paths to Health Equity."[9] The panel was chaired by Michele K. Evans, a biomedical researcher, and in addition to myself, the panelists included Ruth Shim, a cultural psychiatrist; Sarah Tishkoff, a geneticist; and Winifred W. Williams, a transplantation nephrologist. (An audio-recording of the panel is available on the *NEJM* website; see note 9.) Table 11.1 lists the questions addressed to the panel. The panelists were unanimous in stating that genetic differences between human populations do not account for the disparity we observe in complex diseases in the United States and around the world. This is a particularly important and credible consensus given that Sara Tishkoff has published some of the most comprehensive studies of genetic variation in Africans and African Americans.[10] Those studies demolished the typological conception of the "African" and detailed the vast amount of genetic diversity that exists in and between the regions of Africa compared with the rest of the world. The panel also highlighted the importance of expanding the training of medical practitioners to include population genetics and the social determinants of health.

In early 2022, shortly after the publication of *Racism, Not Race*, the book I coauthored with Alan Goodman, Andrea and I published two papers in the high-profile medical journals: the *NEJM* and *Academic Medicine*. The *Academic Medicine* article highlighted ongoing medical misconceptions in medicine.[11] The *NEJM* paper discussed Andrea's comprehensive investigation into the myth of racial differences in keloid formation, specifically that "Black" skin is more likely than white skin to form keloids (thick fibrous scars formed after skin injury) and that 16 percent of people of African descent have keloids. Andrea showed that this figure originated in a non-peer-reviewed article from 1931 that reported keloid incidence in 1,205 Congolese mine workers. By contrast, in the same issue of that journal, another researcher showed that the incidence of keloids in adult Swiss (white) men was 13.3 percent, a difference that may have been statistically significant but certainly lacked clinical significance. Nonetheless, the 16 percent figure spread throughout the medical literature, becoming an established medical "fact" in many resources and reference works, including *UptoDate*, (a database that has been used by clinicians for the last 30 years) that has persisted into the twenty-first century, while the 13.3 percent figure cited in Swiss men was lost to history.[12] Reaction to the *NEJM* article was swift, with keloid experts from around the nation claiming that they had definitive

TABLE 11.1

Questions and responses from the 2021 "Race in Medicine" panel sponsored by the *New England Journal of Medicine*

Question	Respondent(s)	Key points
Is race a social construct?	Graves, Tishkoff	Biological and social conceptions of race are different conceptions; genetic diversity exists in humans but not enough to justify the claim that biological races exist.
How do we use race in the context of the social determinants of health in the United States?	Shim	Race is not a proxy for the social determinants of health.
How is race a risk factor in disease?	Graves, Shim, Williams	Because of structural racism, wealth differences influence health disparities.
How does the lack of workforce diversity impact biomedical research and clinical practice?	Graves, Tishkoff	Lack of diversity contributes to the replication of scientific inaccuracies; medical students should receive population genetics training.
How does the interaction between genes and the environment impact disease?	Graves, Tishkoff	Examples include the *APOL1* locus and end-stage renal disease, evolutionary mismatch, and gene–environment interactions.
What are the panel's recommendations?	All panelists	Stop using race as a proxy for the social determinants of health; the pharmaceutical industry needs more diversity in the participants used in drug trials; we must recognize that genetic differences play only a small role in creating health disparities; we must recognize the influence of structural racism in clinical medicine.

Source: M. K. Evans et al., "Race in Medicine—Genetic Variation, Social Categories, and Paths to Health Equity," *New England Journal of Medicine* 385, no. 14 (2021): e45.

evidence of the statistically significantly greater likelihood of keloid formation in Blacks.[13] For example, a 2011 study that examined keloid formation in 429 patients found that 7.1 percent of Blacks and 0.1 percent of whites had keloids (odds ratio [OR], 16/1), whereas a 2014 study of a much larger group of patients (6,691) found that 0.8 percent of Blacks and 0.1 percent of whites formed keloids (OR, 7/1). The differences in the rates keloid formation between the two studies is already evidence that making the claim of an inherent Black–white difference in keloid formation is flawed. This all underscores that we do not actually have good data on keloid formation across world populations, so making a claim of inherent "racial" difference in this context is unmerited.

Andrea and I worked with two other colleagues to write the *Academic Medicine* article.[14] These included Lainie Ross, a practicing pediatrician and philosopher who was the associate director of the MacLean Center for Clinical Medical Ethics and the co-director of the Institute for Translational Medicine at the University of Chicago, and Lainie's student, Alice Li. This paper examined how the concept of race was manifested in the second edition of the *American Academy of Pediatrics Textbook of Pediatric Care*.[15] We achieved this by searching for twenty-nine race- and ethnicity-related terms on the American Academy of Pediatrics (AAP) e-book platform. We extracted direct quotes containing at least one such term (finding 806) and then examined them to determine whether they were problematic. The problematic quotes were those that (1) used race or ethnicity as a surrogate for social variables; (2) conflated terminology, such as *socially defined race* and *genetic ancestry*; (3) overgeneralized or made claims based on limited data; (4) lacked clinical relevance; (5) lacked inclusivity; (6) promoted racial stereotypes; or (7) made contradicting claims about race. We used the mnemonic "SCORSIC" for these categories. We found that all problematic uses of race- and ethnicity-related terms appeared often, commonly, or abundantly in the text (table 11.2). However, it should be noted that, really, *all* uses of race- and ethnicity-related terms were problematic. In our article, we made a concrete recommendation to researchers and clinicians to always keep the SCORISC categories in mind when engaging in biomedical research. clinical practice, and medical writing.

The paper was first published online on March 15, 2022. On May 2 that year, the AAP released a statement that it was in opposition to racial medicine, which it published in the journal *Pediatrics* in July 2022.[16] However, neither the online press release nor the paper published in *Pediatrics* cited our paper. It is possible that the AAP had already planned to come out publicly against racial medicine before our paper brought the errors in their text to light, though I doubt it. But what is most important is that they did make the statement. Though we need more professional medical associations to make statements against racial medicine, more important is to embed education and training to eliminate racial misconceptions in undergraduate education, medical school admissions testing, medical school training, and ongoing professional training.

TABLE 11.2

Problematic Uses of Race and Ethnicity in the *American Academy of Pediatrics Textbook of Pediatric Care, 2nd Edition*[20]

Category[a]	Questions asked (if yes to any, then use considered problematic)[b]	Examples[b]
Using race as a *surrogate* for social variables	Does the statement use race as a biologically valid category?	Other factors that may predict smoking include peer influence, lower socioeconomic status, psychiatric and substance abuse disorders, Alaskan native and Native American ethnicity, and military service. (p. 2282)
	Does the statement highlight differences between races without correcting for education, socioeconomic status, rural/urban, single-parent home, or other factors?	[Box 298-3] Criteria for Screening High-Risk Children for Diabetes: [second bullet point] High-risk race or ethnicity (Native American, African American, Latino, Asian American, and Pacific Islander). (p. 2402)
Conflating terminology	Does the statement use terms interchangeably for socially defined race, ancestry, and skin color?	Racial differences [in cleft lip or palate] are seen in incidence, with children of Asian descent having a higher incidence (2.1 in 1,000) and those of African descent having a lower incidence (0.41 in 1,000) compared with white children (1.3 in 1,000). (p. 1850–1851) [This statement also lacks clinical relevance.]
		The risk for severe hyperbilirubinemia is increased in infants of East Asian descent and decreased in black infants. Correct identification of race and ethnicity by asking the mother about the maternal and paternal ancestry is important in assessing the risk to an infant. (p. 859)
Overgeneralizing or making claims based on limited data	Does the statement make an overgeneralization about a large group?	Overall, no racial differences were noted, but a subset analysis showed an increased proportion of white infants with Ebstein anomaly, aortic stenosis, coarctation of the aorta, transposition of the great vessels, and pulmonary atresia. (p. 888)
	Does the statement draw a conclusion about racial differences based on a study with limited internal or external validity?	[Table 69-2] Biomedical Conditions in the Health Care of Children That Can Result from Harmful Folk Illness Remedies or Parental Beliefs and Practices. (p. 582)
		Regional origin: Latin America
		Condition: Gonococcal conjunctivitis Associated folk illness, parental belief, or symptom: Conjunctivitis Ethnicity or nationality that may have folk illness or parental belief: Latinos Harmful treatment associated with condition: Adult urine as treatment for conjunctivitis in children
		Culturally acceptable alternative folk treatments: Special diet: vegetable soup and fresh fruits, carrot juice, eliminate flour tortillas, bread, soda

(*continued*)

TABLE 11.2
(continued)

Category[a]	Questions asked (if yes to any, then use considered problematic)	Examples[b]
Lacking clinical *relevance*	Does the statement present epidemiological data in which there is such little difference between racial groups that clinical relevance is minimal?	In an American study, agenesis of the third molars was more common in white than in black adolescents (16% vs 6%) and slightly more common in females than in males (19% vs 14%). (p. 1949) Racial and ethnic variations can be found in birth weight, with non-Hispanic white and Hispanic infants having higher mean birth weights than non-Hispanic black infants. Mean (±1 standard deviation) birth weights were reported as 3,375g (±554), 3,316g (±548), and 3,115g (±628) for non-Hispanic white, Hispanic, and non-Hispanic black infants, respectively. (p. 804–805)
Lacking *inclusivity*	Does the statement focus on only 1 or 2 groups without mentioning others?	Acrocyanosis, blue color of the hands and feet when the rest of the body is pink, is frequently seen in newborns. (p. 869)
	Is there an assumption of a particular skin tone?	Infantile hemangiomas develop in 1.1 % to 2.6% of newborns; incidence figures at the end of 1 year are 10% to 12% of white infants. The prevalence is highest in low-birth-weight, white, female infants. (p. 821)
Promoting racial *stereotypes*	Does the statement promote racial stereotypes or assume homogeneity within a population?	[Chapter 302: Oppositional Defiant Disorder] Case Report: Keenan, a 9-year-old African American boy, arrives for his annual well-child with his mother . . . (p. 2427) Although the dominant American culture values stoicism and nonemotional expressions of pain, other cultures may express pain through screaming, moaning, and verbal complaining. (p. 339)
Making *contradicting* claims about race	Is the statement inconsistent with other statements in the text?	Native American children suffer significantly more infections from RMSF [Rocky Mountain spotted fever] than other ethnic groups. (p. 2312) The illness [RMSF] occurs more frequently in boys than girls and more in white people than people of other races. (p. 2593) No evidence has been found demonstrating large genetic differences in birth weight among various populations; thus the use of separate, race-specific reference curves, even in situations in which race is associated with other risk factors such as poor nutrition or low socioeconomic status, is not supported. (p. 804) Race and ethnicity also play an important role [in intrauterine growth restriction]. The growth curves should ideally be tailored to the patient population and geographic region. (p. 848)

[a] The authors developed the SCORISC mnemonic to identify the questions that need to be asked to determine whether race, ethnicity, and ancestry are being used correctly in medical writing. The words used in the mnemonic appear in italics.

[b] Quotes are copied verbatim from the *American Academy of Pediatrics Textbook of Pediatric Care, 2nd Edition* using the capitalization and word choices of the original authors.

FAITH OF THE MUSTARD SEED

In the book of Matthew (13:31–32), Christ refers to the kingdom of heaven as a mustard seed. He explains that while it is the smallest of seeds, when planted, it grows to become one of the biggest trees in the garden. Social change can also be viewed as a mustard seed. My brother, Warren (1957–1997), was someone who went into medicine because he wanted to help people. We were the children of poor African Americans growing up during the civil rights movement. We lived the reality of health disparity. Our parents could not afford to provide us regular visits to the doctor. We received no dental care unless a tooth had become infected and needed extraction. We watched our uncles and aunts die before their time. So, for Warren, medical school meant making a difference in the lives of oppressed people. I have observed this sentiment in disproportionate numbers of the Black and Brown students whom I have mentored and for whom I have written letters of recommendation for health-related careers.

Not everyone pursues a career in medicine to help people or to "make the world a better place." Some go into the profession because they find it intrinsically interesting. Others do it for the lucrative salary. For others, it feeds some aspect of cravings for power and prestige. Social dominance orientation (SDO) is a measure of the comfort and desire a person has for advancing in social hierarchy. SDO has been measured across a variety of professions. It is low in professions devoted to helping people, such as social workers, teachers, and paramedics, and high in politicians, bankers, corporate administrators, police officers, and prison guards. In the United States, it is generally higher in males than females and generally higher in whites than nonwhites.[17] Measurements of SDO show a clear relationship between that trait and the desire to pursue specialty training in medical school.[18] There has been no comprehensive analysis of the distribution of SDO in medicine, but it is clearly variable and undoubtedly has an influence on the willingness of individuals to engender or tolerate change in the profession. In the past, medical students were predominantly male, but that have shifted so that now the gender of medical school trainees is more balanced.[19] However, a negative correlation still exists between medical schools' research ranking and the percentage of female medical trainees at those schools.[20]

Because of Andrea's role in revising *Robbins Basic Pathology* and her many professional contacts in the fields of pathology and medical education, the two of us began lecturing at medical schools and hospitals across the United States, Canada, and the United Kingdom in 2022 (table 11.3).

TABLE 11.3
Deyrup and Graves: selected medical lectures, 2021–2024

Department	Institutions
Pathology	Duke University, University of California – Los Angeles, University of California – San Francisco, University of Pittsburgh, University of Minnesota, University of Vermont, Harvard University, Creighton University, Yale University, Stanford University, Ohio State University, University of Chicago, Eastern Carolina University, Emory University, University of Virginia, Johns Hopkins University, University of Southern California, Uniformed Services University of the Health Sciences, University of New Mexico, Georgetown University, Memorial Sloan Kettering Cancer Center, Montefiore Medical Center
Pediatrics	Duke University, John Hopkins University, University of Virginia, Our Lady of the Lake Health, Nicklaus Children's Hospital
Medical Education	Duke University, Vanderbilt Academy for Educational Excellence, Harvard–MIT Health Sciences and Technology, Campbell University School of Medicine, Georgetown University Interdisciplinary, UC Davis Medical School, National Board Medical Education Invitational Conference for Educators, Group Research in Pathology Education
Critical Care	Mount Sinai Hospital, New York City
Evolutionary Medicine Summer Institute	MDs, PhDs, graduate students, and medical students worldwide
Medical Oncology	Memorial Sloan Kettering Cancer Center
Others	Duke University departments of Clinical Research, Dermatology, Family Medicine, Neurology, Ophthalmology, and Radiology.
Miscellaneous	National Board of Medical Examiners (NBME), NBME Invitational Conference for Educators, American Board of Pathology, National Board of Osteopathic Medical Educators, College of American Pathologists and American Medical Association diversity committees

These talks are an evolving lecture crafted by Andrea titled variously "Race in *Robbins*: Data or Distraction" and "(Nearly) Everything You Learned About Race in Medical School Is Wrong." The objectives of the lectures are to discuss the impact of systemic racism in health professions' curricula, compare and contrast biological race with socially defined race, evaluate disparities in the pathophysiology of disease, and describe an approach to addressing health disparities in health care education.[21] Andrea explains that the tenth edition of *Robbins Basic Pathology* discusses thirty-eight health disparities, of which twenty-one are described as being more prevalent or having worse prognoses in Blacks and only seven are similarly described in whites. This narrative contributes to the mythology of the inherently sick Black person as opposed to the notion that Blacks are being made sick by the cumulative impact of structural racism.[22] This narrative also has a chilling impact on Black medical students, as described by Damon Tweedy in his book *Black Man in a White Coat*: "It seemed that no matter the body part or organ system affected, the [medical school] lecturers would sound a familiar refrain: 'It's more common in Blacks than in whites.'"[23]

My role in Andrea's and my lecture series is to provide scientific data demonstrating the differences between biological and social conceptions of race and to explain why biological race does not exist in modern humans. I also discuss admixture so that the physicians will better understand the differences between subpopulations in the African diaspora and among Latin Americans. Latin Americans comprise groups created by colonization and slavery in the Western Hemisphere beginning in 1492. Their genetic profiles vary greatly, displaying a combination of African, Amerindian, and European ancestry.[24] For example, the two largest groups of Latinos (or Hispanics) in the United States are Mexican Americans and Puerto Ricans. Mexican Americans have an average ancestry profile of 51 percent Amerindian, 46 percent European (mostly from the Iberian Peninsula), and 3 percent African, whereas Puerto Ricans are on average 16 percent Amerindian, 72 percent European (mostly from the Iberian Peninsula), and 12 percent African. Yet in all Latin American nations, subgroups exist with dramatically different ancestry profiles from the national average, such as in the state of Chocó in Colombia. Colombia's national average ancestry profile is 29 percent Amerindian, 64 percent European, and 7 percent African, but in Chocó, which was a site of gold mining, an industry that used large numbers of enslaved Africans, the ancestry profile is on average about 80 percent African.[25] But the people living in Chocó see themselves as Colombians; they become racialized as "white" or "Black" only when they emigrate to the United States.

We then go on to familiarize the audience with the social determinants of health as a means to help them address implicit racial bias. We discuss the differences between individual acts of racism and institutional and systemic or structural racism. We find that many physicians are aware of individual acts of racism but have thought much less about institutional and structural racism in society at large and how it manifests in medicine. We illustrate this by examining some widely held but false beliefs in medicine, such as that Blacks experience a greater prevalence of keloids. We also provide examples of differences in disease prevalence that have no clinical relevance in differential diagnosis. We then discuss the importance of inclusive images in medical texts. Finally, we call on physicians who wish to redress the harm caused by racial medicine to form teams of like-minded individuals to address how race is addressed in their curricula and medical practices.

It is difficult to evaluate how much progress we have made on the lecture circuit over the past three years. We have some unpublished data demonstrating that physicians' understanding of biological and social conceptions of race improve after hearing the lecture. The talks are usually well attended, and discussions afterward are usually spirited, indicating that many audience members have been paying attention and want to make change. However, there are also clear signs of resistance. For example, in March 2024, Andrea and I were asked to speak at the 113th Annual Meeting of the United States and Canadian Society of Pathology (USCAP). We were joined by the statistical geneticist and genetic epidemiologist Genevieve Wojcik from Johns Hopkins University. Dr. Wojcik served on the committee that drafted a report on population descriptors commissioned by the National Academies of Science, Engineering, and Medicine.[26] The USCAP meeting is the largest meeting of pathologists in the world. However, our session was scheduled for 8 A.M. on the morning of Palm Sunday, and virtually no one was in the room before our presentation began aside from the panelists. The presidents of two societies supporting the meeting made an appearance before the session started but did not stay for the presentation. A few others made their way into the room after we began speaking, but at most only about twenty people attended. However, the lecture was recorded, and to date more than 331 people have since viewed the recording and left comments, such as the following: "Very thought-provoking and relevant course. I really enjoyed this and learned new ways to approach doing and evaluating research," and "This was one of the most interesting and valuable conferences that I listened to."

I had a similar experience at the American Society of Hematology Annual Meeting and Exposition in December 2024. Each year, about two thousand to three thousand physicians attend the meeting. I was invited to participate in a symposium titled "Race, Structural Racism and the Social Determinants of Health in Hematology." It was also scheduled early in the morning, and though the room could have held three hundred people, we had about thirty attendees. Race was clearly a topic of interest for the society as a search of the conference program using the keyword "race" returned hits for more than three hundred sessions that had something to do with the topic. However, upon reviewing these sessions, I saw that socially defined race was being used in the same ways that my colleagues and I had critiqued in our *Academic Medicine* paper.

Professional societies make clear what their priorities are at their national and international meetings. At USCAP, featured lectures addressed molecular testing in pathology and human genomics. Such lectures are scheduled so as not to conflict with any other programming and are held at prime time; in this case, each was held at 5 P.M. (on separate days). Our presentation was not listed by name in the online program; rather, it was ambiguously titled "American Society of Clinical Pathology."[27] Further, it was held at one of the worst possible times in the schedule, 8 A.M. on a Sunday, and was run concurrently with eight other sessions. Interestingly, the USCAP program committee had been enthusiastic about our session proposal and had accepted it immediately. However, the impact of our session was definitely negatively impacted by the poor scheduling.

This is just another example of how covert resistance to effecting change in scientific and medical societies operates, especially when supporters of the status quo see the efforts of those from nondominant groups (e.g., racialized people, LGBTQ+ people, women) as "political correctness" as opposed to efforts to improve scientific accuracy in the service of improving patient care. The "mustard seed" challenge that we face is that the medical profession is still dominated by whites in numbers disproportionate to their representation in their nations' populations. According to the most recent data, only about 5.7 percent of American physicians are Black, though Blacks compose 13 percent of the national population.[28] Disproportionate representation is particularly egregious in leadership positions, where nonwhites are dramatically underrepresented, particularly by gender.[29] The demography of the physician workforce has impacts on patient outcomes. For example, physician identity plays a critical role in reducing mortality in nonwhite patients.[30] Things will be made worse over the coming years by the Supreme Court's decision to strike down affirmative action in college admissions at all levels. This means that fewer Black and Brown students will be admitted to America's elite and historically white medical schools. Indeed, a recent report from the Association of American Medical Colleges shows that in 2024, there were drops of 11.6 and 10.8 percent in the enrollment of Black and Hispanic students in American medical schools, respectively, because of the dismissal of affirmative action.[31] I predict that without significant numbers of nonwhite physicians in the medical professions, the fallacies of racial medicine will get worse, not better. Thus, it is imperative that physicians committed to racial justice intensify their efforts to make curricular changes that undo the racial misconceptions with which students enter medical schools and to resist all forms of discrimination against Black and Brown students in medical school admissions and recruitment into medical professions.

TOWARD AN ANTI-RACIST CURRICULUM

Racist ideology relies on the suppositions that biological races exist in our species and that these races are genetically different in meaningful ways.[32] These ways include behavior, intelligence, and disease predisposition. Biological racism was actively taught in American science curricula until the 1960s.[33] The civil rights movement resulted in the retreat of overt racism in scientific research and teaching, but it was never completely defeated. From the latter half of the twentieth century to the present, a key problem has been the benign neglect of curricula that address human biological variation meaningfully. This has resulted in students graduating from high school and institutions of higher education with false beliefs about human biological variation. This is evidenced by national polls concerning biological race, genetic determinism, and human evolution.[34] It is clear how these beliefs came about, and it is clear that our education system is doing nothing to dispel them.

More than twenty years ago, I wrote an essay for the *Reports of the National Center for Science Education* explaining why we should teach students about race in the K–12 curriculum. I reprised this argument with even more emphasis in 2023 for the *American Biology Teacher*.[35] Three major problems stand in the way of developing such curricula. The first is historic. To effectively teach about human variation and biological conceptions of race, you must teach human evolution. This is difficult to achieve in many areas of the nation owing to special creationist opposition to teaching evolution in the K–12 grades. The second is also historic: K–12 teachers have not been well prepared to teach evolution.[36] Since 1982, the National Center for Science Education (of which I am a board member) has been working to provide teachers with lesson plans to help them more effectively dismiss students' misconceptions about evolution (and now also climate change).[37] However, despite the hard work of its staff, its efforts to support teachers have been limited, particularly in the states with the highest proportions of underserved Black and Brown students.[38]

The third and newest problem standing in the way of teaching about race in K–12 is the association of such teaching with what is now often referred to pejoratively as "wokeness." On June 5, 2021, Donald Trump delivered his first public address outside Florida after leaving office following his first administration to the North Carolina Republican Party State Convention.[39] During that speech, he felt compelled to address the topic of critical race theory three times. About three minutes into the speech, he claimed that the Biden administration was pushing "toxic" critical race theory. He returned to this theme about forty-five minutes later, referring to critical race theory as a divisive left-wing doctrine and calling on Republicans at all levels to move for legislation banning the teaching of critical race theory in public schools.[40] Trump's call found willing adherents, and soon after laws attacking critical race theory were penned across the nation in twenty-eight states. By June 17, 2021, five states (Idaho, Iowa, Oklahoma, Tennessee, and Texas) had passed anti–critical race theory legislation. In Tennessee, the Republican governor, Bill Lee, signed into law a measure that withholds funding from school districts if teachers tie certain events to institutional racism, white privilege, or critical race theory. House Bill 11 in Alabama declared, "The Alabama Board of Education believes that the United States of America is not an inherently racist country, and the state of Alabama is not an inherently racist state."[41] Of course, critical race theory does not claim that any country or state is "inherently" racist. It claims that the much of the history of the United States has been driven by racist ideology. These are very different statements.

Further complicating the problem is the Supreme Court's June 2023 decision to strike down affirmative action in higher education. This has led to historically white institutions across the nation, particularly those in formerly Confederate states, dismantling diversity, equity, and inclusion (DEI) programs. For example, on April 2, 2024, the University of Texas at Austin fired forty-nine staffers associated with DEI.[42] The connection between programs that affirm DEI and curricula that address why we should be promoting DEI has always been strong. Thus, striking down these programs in higher education sends a message to K–12 educators about the value of course work addressing structural racism and social definitions of race. Under these conditions, I predict that teaching about these topics and any student learning associated with them in K–12 will get worse, not better. These political developments are truly unfortunate, especially given the progress that has been made in producing tools that can be used in K–12 programming to reduce misconceptions about genetic determinism and counter racism. The work of Brian Donovan and his colleagues is particularly relevant in this regard.[43] And one reason that Alan Goodman and I wrote *Racism, Not Race* was to provide K–12 teachers with easily accessible information to help them more effectively teach about human biological variation and social conceptions of race.[44]

At the university level, more can be achieved to challenge the racial misconceptions that many students entering the health professions bring with
them. Currently, only students who take courses in biological anthropology,
or who are lucky enough to take their genetics and evolution coursework
with professors who understand the importance of teaching about racial
misconceptions and human biological variation, will encounter this material. However, the vast majority of undergraduate students never take such
courses. For example, the chemistry students that I mentor in the University of North Carolina Greensboro's Maximizing Access to Research Careers
(MARC) program (see chapter 10) typically have no exposure to human
evolutionary and population genetics until the workshops I give in the program every summer.

Performance on the Medical College Admission Test (MCAT) plays a
significant role in determining who goes to medical school. There is no evidence of implicit racial bias in the MCAT, at least by standard measures.[45]
The test doesn't assess medical knowledge but rather general science knowledge and some sociology, so there is likely little, if any, racial medicine in its
questions. (I have not taken the MCAT myself.) However, medical licensing
exams do contain the racial misconceptions that are still prevalent among
US physicians.[46] Thus, Andrea and I have argued for racialized questions
to be removed from the high-stakes exams involved in the progression of
medical professionals.

To address the ongoing problem of racial misconceptions in the training of
physicians and other health professionals, schools should require that students
take at least one upper-level course in biological anthropology; in evolutionary,
population, or quantitative genetics; or that addresses the social determinants
of health. And curriculum committees should be charged with examining
course content to determining equivalencies in content across courses.

This would not be difficult to achieve. Of course, I often hear the argument that adding material addressing racial misconceptions to medical
school curricula is too difficult because curricula are already overwhelmed
with content. But this is not a valid argument. The lack of attention to human
variation in medical training and clinical practice is a clear problem that will
only grow larger as the next generation of pharmacogenomic results becomes
integrated into treatment options for patients. The lack of understanding of
modern human biological diversity has significant impacts on patients from
historically underserved populations that contribute to poorer treatment
outcomes compared with whites. So, it comes down to the question of what

the priorities of medical training are. If equity and justice are valued, then content that advances those aims should be added to curricula. This could be achieved by adding material to existing courses (as Andrea as done in her pathology course) or by creating new courses.

However, there is resistance to addressing ongoing racial misconceptions in medicine. In March 2024, with the support of forty cosponsors, the Republican congressman Greg Murphy (representing the Third District of North Carolina) introduced a bill to cut off federal funding to medical schools that force students to adopt "specific beliefs, discriminate based on race or ethnicity, or have diversity, equity, or inclusion (DEI) offices or functional equivalences."[47] As of the time of this writing, the bill has not been voted on by Congress. Of course, curricular content that explains to medical students why human biological variation does not align with social conceptions of race does not force anyone to "believe" anything, just as teaching the function of the kidney doesn't force anyone to adopt a particular belief. Science is a system based on testing hypotheses, and it is always conjectural, based on the best available evidence. However, it is the goal of Murphy and his allies to characterize science that eliminates racial misconceptions as a system of DEI-based indoctrination. We cannot allow this argument to win the day.

Given the current political climate, I have argued that historically Black colleges and universities and minority-serving institutions have an oversized role to play in producing the next generation of Black and Brown scholars in science and medicine.[48] However, these institutions are crippled by historical and ongoing underfunding. My own university has been underfunded by more than $2 billion since 1930.[49] This is a problem across the former Confederate states, which have systematically diverted funds away from Black education to pay for white education. These funds were guaranteed under the Supreme Court's 1896 *Plessy v. Ferguson* ruling, which allowed segregation in public facilities as long as the facilities were funded equally.[50] In 2021, the State of Maryland agreed to pay a settlement of $577 million for the historical and systematic underfunding of its four historically Black colleges and universities.[51] Restorative justice has not yet been brought to the other states that conducted this unjust practice. Yet I argue that all citizens of these states, not just Black and Brown people, should be calling on their legislatures to restore the funding withheld from their historically Black colleges and universities and minority-serving institutions. This would be a gigantic step forward in increasing the number of Black and Brown people in a variety of professions, not just medicine and science. This is justice that cannot wait.

CONCLUSION

Building a World Where We Can All Live Well

The primary message of this book is that medicine has historically gotten race wrong and continues to do so. This is true in both biomedical research and clinical practice. I argue this happens because most people in health professions come to their careers with attitudes and ideologies formed by societies that never questioned their understanding of the concepts of race, both biological and social. This is also true of individuals who have been oppressed by social conceptions of race. Racial misconceptions in medicine persist in part because of the historical and ongoing underdevelopment of educational institutions—from kindergarten through medical school. I know this is the case because I teach courses in genetics, evolution, health disparities, and biological and social definitions of race at North Carolina Agricultural and Technical State University, the nation's largest historically Black postsecondary institution. Students who take my courses have virtually no background in these disciplines. They enter with many of the same racial misconceptions that I witnessed in white, Hispanic, and Native American students when I taught these subjects at historically white R1 institutions (i.e., those with very high research activity), such as the University of California, Irvine, and Arizona State University. And though they are more likely than students at historically white institutions to accept that humans first evolved in Africa, they can provide no logical argument for why this is true.[1]

The second reason that medicine has persistently gotten race wrong is its historical lack of appreciation of evolutionary biology. Theodosius

Dobzhansky, one of the foremost minds of the neo-Darwinian synthesis, once said, "Nothing in biology makes sense, except in the light of evolution."[2] The truth of this statement has been demonstrated repeatedly over the last fifty years in subject areas ranging from antibiotic resistance and the prevalence of genetic diseases to the evolution of aging. Yet biomedical research and clinical practice have often proceeded without reference to this powerful dictum. This is a theme I carried throughout this book, particularly in parts I and II. The significance of evolutionary thinking to medicine was prominently announced to the world with the publication of Randolph Nesse and George C. Williams's popular book *Why We Get Sick* in 1994.[3] Nesse is a practicing psychiatrist and Williams (1926–2010) was an evolutionary biologist who helped shape much of our modern understanding of adaptation. Believing that an understanding of evolutionary thinking could improve biomedical research and clinical practice, Nesse brought together scholars from the fields of biological anthropology, evolutionary biology, and medicine, including me, to found the International Society for Evolution, Medicine & Public Health (ISEMPH) in 2014. Throughout 2015, I participated in a series of workshops attempting to communicate the importance of evolutionary thinking to medical practitioners. The working group included physicians from the Association of American Medical Colleges, the University of Auckland, Harvard University, the Institute of Medicine (now the National Academy of Medicine), the University of Kansas Medical Center, the University of Michigan, New York University, Pennsylvania State University, the University of California at Los Angeles, and Yale University.[4] During one session the dean of medicine at Duke University attended.

Yet even within the evolutionary medicine community, there was little appreciation for how evolutionary theory correctly explained racial health disparities. Nor was there a uniform understanding of the difference between the biological and social definitions of race. At international ISEMPH meetings, I often found myself sitting through research presentations in which the presenters spouted the same typological logic about race that I could have heard at any American medical school. For this reason, I went to work explaining to the evolutionary medicine community how ongoing racial misconceptions were holding back the usefulness of the field.[5] But despite these efforts over the last decade, the significance of the evolutionary approach to understanding disease, health disparities, and lifespan is still not widely appreciated in evolutionary medicine or in medicine as a whole. A 2023 paper I coauthored on this topic was one of the most read in the journal *Evolution, Medicine, and Public Health*.[6] These facts are evidence that we have much work to do going forward to bring together a coherent biomedical research program to improve patient care and eliminate health disparities.

SOCIAL DETERMINANTS OF HEALTH, NOT GENES

Throughout this book, I have made the case that it is the social determinants of health—not genetic differences—that drive the health disparities we observe in American society. In chapters 3, 5, 6, 7, and 8, I presented this argument for diseases with both simple and complex genetic foundations. Evolutionary genetic theory shows that diseases with simple genetics (e.g., cystic fibrosis, sickle cell anemia) will be found at various frequencies across world populations because of the combined action of natural selection and genetic drift; distribution is not predicted simply by socially defined race. For example, cystic fibrosis is found worldwide, but because of population admixture (which occurred during the time of slavery), it is found at higher frequencies in African Americans than in West Africans. The failure of American physicians to understand that has often led to problems diagnosing and treating the disease in African Americans.[7] Diseases with complex foundations, such as cancer and heart disease, also differ in prevalence by socially defined race.

Genome-wide association studies have found common genetic markers for diseases and some that are unique by population; however, genetic differences in populations do not drive health disparities either. Indeed, what we know about the genomics of disease-causing variants suggests that it is whites—not Blacks—who should experience higher rates of simple and complex diseases. An early study of disease risk variants examined those that were possibly "bad" and those that were probably "bad." Black and white Americans did not differ significantly in the frequency of variants that were possibly bad, but whites were statistically significantly more likely than Blacks to have a genetic variant that was probably bad.[8] Not much can be made from that study because it evaluated only fifteen Black and twenty white genomes. However, in February 2024, the All of Us Research Program released a study of more than 245,000 clinical-grade genomes. The authors found that genomes of European ancestry had more pathogenic and likely pathogenic variants than did genomes of African and American Indian ancestry.[9] Data like this do much to challenge claims that health disparities in complex diseases result from genetic differences between socially defined racial groups. Indeed, the genomic data suggests that we should see the *opposite* pattern from what we observe; that is, we should see higher rates of mortality from heart disease, cancer, and stroke in whites than in Blacks. Modern omics research in epigenetics has also revealed the role of non-nucleotide based changes as causal agents in these diseases. Epigenetic changes are also markers of present and past environmental exposures, further driving home the importance of the physical and social environment in determining patterns of disease.

While we should never stop trying to improve how we treat complex diseases, growing evidence suggests that the costs of new technologies may actually exacerbate health disparities (see chapters 9 and 10). This notion raises the question of how much we as a society are committed to reducing and eliminating health disparities. If we are indeed committed, then the immediate solutions will not be found in research to develop new treatments. I have been saying this for over twenty years.[10] Throughout this book, I have explained that a combination of genetic, physical environmental, and social environmental factors operate to greatly reduce how long people live.

Yet the promise of new technologies that will improve our health should not be considered without thinking about how their benefits will be distributed. Our history provides us with a clear answer: wealthy people, who in the United States are disproportionately white, will be the ones to benefit most from new technologies. The Black–white health disparities we observe today began on slave ships. The disparities were then perpetuated throughout the social institutions of chattel slavery, the Jim Crow era, and today's era of mass incarceration. These institutions did not come into existence by chance, or by the will of God. Human beings chose to implement them.

Consider what our racial and ethnic health profiles would look like now if we had collectively made different choices in the past. What would we see today if, in 1691, Virginia had not passed a law differentiating white from Black indentured servants. The latter were made slaves for life, could be bought and sold, and lost all rights to their own bodies and those of their children. The former were able to work their way out of servitude. Our medical views of Black people were born in a society that manifested injustice at all levels. What profile would we see today if Andrew Jackson and his allies had not forced the five civilized tribes off their land in the Carolinas, Georgia, and Tennessee? Would Native American men have such high rates of substance abuse, and rank second in the nation for mortality by suicide, if Europeans had learned to live with their ancestors them in peace? What profile would we see today if Andrew Johnson had not resisted Reconstruction and if the 4.5 million freed Blacks had been given land and the education to pursue skilled trades and professions such as law, medicine, and science? Wouldn't the economy of the former Confederate states have recovered more quickly? Wouldn't those states have avoided the smallpox epidemics that broke out first among displaced former slaves before spreading to whites? What would we see today if the Southern Democrats ("Dixiecrats") had allowed Franklin Roosevelt to pass the New Deal with provisions to serve the needs of agricultural and domestic workers? What would we see today if the value of Black homes had not been undervalued by the practice of redlining? The early progress of the COVID-19 pandemic was linked to the crowed housing conditions created by historical redlining (see chapter 5). What would we see if residential segregation had not created communities where families do not have ready access to healthy foods? What would we see if equal funding for education had been made available for all American children instead of funding being based on property values? Education level is one the most consistent indicators of health in the United States.[11] These are all examples of social and political choices that the ruling classes of American society made to benefit themselves at the cost of the health of racialized others. These are also choices that did not have to be made. Capitalism as an economic system would have worked fine or even better, some argue, if more equitable and just choices had been made.

Because of our nation's history, effective strategies to address health disparities cannot be made in isolation from efforts to dismantle structural racism. Capitalism and racism were joined at the hip at birth. Some argue that there is no way to dismantle racism without also dismantling capitalism.[12] Whether or not that is true, things can be done now to make our society more just. In chapter 11 of *Racism, Not Race*, Alan Goodman and I lay out a series of recommendations on how to begin this process. These include taking action to remove injustices in voting and elections, policing, employment opportunities, the education system, and the health care system. With regard to health care, removing injustices involves adopting universal health care and rapidly expanding the training and licensing of physicians and physician assistants to include more people from historically underrepresented and underserved communities. As in chapter 11 of this book, we also called for the expansion of medical school curricula to include content that teaches human biological variation in the context of clinical care.[13]

THINGS MIGHT GET WORSE BEFORE THEY GET BETTER

The social process of making choices that differentially harm some and help others is ongoing. With every new technology introduced, we have contributed to creating more disease related to evolutionary mismatch. During World War II, per- and polyfluoroalkylated compounds (PFASs) were created to waterproof machinery. These compounds undoubtedly helped save lives at the front and eventually win the war. However, after the war, these compounds were used to create labor-saving nonstick cookware, products that were mass-marketed even after studies in lab animals had demonstrated that they could cause cancer.[14] The industry knew of the dangers of PFAS inhalation and ingestion at least forty years before they were made public. Fast food is another institution that came into existence without a consideration of the potentially serious consequences of its expansion. It began in California in the 1950s with a few hot dog and burger stands. Now it is a global enterprise. Americans spent about $6 billion on fast food in 1970; by 2000, they were spending more than $110 billion. As a nation, we spend more on fast food than higher education, personal computers, computer software, and cars. We spend more on fast food than movies, books, magazines, newspapers, videos, and recorded music combined.[15]

The diseases of evolutionary mismatch (e.g., heart disease, cancer, metabolic syndrome) are being disproportionately shouldered by poor, nonwhite people.[16] Yet these people have little to no say in whether toxic products are introduced into society. Black people did not create menthol cigarettes, and they do not design the racially targeted cigarette and alcohol ads that bombard their communities.[17] Nor where they responsible for flooding heroin into the country in the 1960s, cocaine in the 1980s, or fentanyl in the 2010s. Yet Black and Brown communities suffered the most from these events because of a well-established relationship between social status and substance abuse, a relationship that has also been established in primate models.[18] Research shows that people who are lower in a social hierarchy are more vulnerable to substance use and addiction. This fact partially accounts for the opioid epidemic that differentially affected unemployed white working-class Americans in the last decade.[19] Food addiction is also likely associated with social status given that the same parts of the brain that respond to opiates and other drugs are activated by sweet and fatty foods.

It also plays a role in the relationship between environmental factors, social status, and obesity.[20]

Climate change is another factor that will contribute to growing health disparities. Twenty years ago, the Congressional Black Caucus released a report on the unequal burden that Black communities will face with climate change.[21] Hurricane Katrina, which hit the Gulf Coast in the summer of 2005, flooded 80 percent of New Orleans. Low-income and predominantly Black residents were hardest hit. Most of them were left without a workable plan for escape and no rescue, emergency health services, or shelter. The highest death rate in the immediate wake of the hurricane was in the Ninth Ward, where 90 percent of the residents were Black.[22] The number of powerful hurricanes and tornadoes has been increasing over the last twenty years, and climate models predict a continued increase.[23] Hurricane Beryl, a category 5 storm that hit the Caribbean in late June and early July, 2024, is the earliest-forming category 5 hurricane since records began to be kept about one hundred years ago. In addition to catastrophic storms, the United States has also experienced an increase in extreme heat. The summer of 2023 displayed the hottest temperatures on record, and 2024 overtook them.[24] As I write, the East Coast is under a heat dome, with daily temperatures exceeding 90°F and heat indexes exceeding 100°F. Heat mortality can be caused by heat stroke and dehydration. The most vulnerable populations, which are the same groups at greatest risk from extreme storms, are the elderly, young children, outdoor workers, those who are socially isolated, those who are economically disadvantaged, people experiencing homelessness, those with chronic illnesses and disabilities, those who abuse substances, and urban dwellers.[25] Climate change will also expand the distribution of vector-borne diseases such as Zika virus and malaria (see chapter 5). In 2023, the transmission of malaria (caused by the *Plasmodium vivax* parasite) was documented in Florida and Texas.[26] Given the climates of those areas of the country, it is highly likely that the mosquitoes that are the vectors for *Plasmodium vivax* are already successfully reproducing all over the southeastern United States.

As with significant decisions in our nation's past, the decision to take action to eliminate health disparities is one that we must make collectively. But I am skeptical that we can do so in our current political situation. The two major political parties have very different views about whether addressing health disparities should be a priority. The Democrats have talked a good game but have really made little progress on this issue. And the Republicans have branded themselves the "party of white people" since 1968.[27] There is nothing in the Trump platform that provides any evidence that his administration will take on this problem. Indeed, it was his lack of attention to the nation's health that accounted for the unnecessary deaths we experienced during the COVID-19 pandemic (see chapter 5). The Republican Party also has a history of acting against programs that would improve the health of all Americans, including the white working-class people who make up much of their base; for example, it opposed *Roe v. Wade* and the Affordable Care Act.[28] Both Democrats and Republicans have failed to effectively confront health disparities because both parties are wedded to the socioeconomic system at the root of the United States: racial capitalism. The Democrats believe that the best way to run this system is by allowing a reasonably sized social welfare safety net to take care of those most dispossessed by the system. Conversely, the Republicans think that the best way to run the system is to use a program of "smoke and mirrors" to convince the white working class that it is Black, Hispanic, and new immigrant populations that are the cause of all their troubles. The Economic Policy Institute has elegantly demonstrated how this strategy continues to contribute to the South's underperforming economy.[29]

As the result of our failed political leadership, we are a nation staggering toward its own doom. The attack on the Capitol on January 6, 2021, was a poorly heeded warning. Few of those responsible for spreading the lies of massive election fraud have ever been brought to justice—including the lead conspirator, Donald J. Trump. Trump and his allies have used a clever program of judicial maneuvering to avoid his being tried or sentenced for crimes associated with his candidacy for the presidency in 2016 and his attempts to overturn the lawful presidential election of 2020. He has turned his criminal behavior into strengths, resulting in his party skillfully placing itself in a position to win the 2024 election. Indeed, the attempted assassination of Trump at a rally in Pennsylvania on July 13, 2024, played a major role in galvanizing his base and helped to deliver him the election. Upon his election he has engaged in an unprecedented grab of political power within the executive branch and unleashed an attack on higher education, including freezing the federal funds of premier institutions such as Columbia, Penn, and Harvard.

These events are eerie reflections of Germany just before Hitler gained the chancellorship. In the Munich Beer Hall Putsch of November 1923, Hitler and the Nazi Party attempted to overthrow the German government. During the incident, police fired on the crowd, narrowly missing Hitler by inches. Hitler was tried for treason but skillfully used the trial to discredit the authorities that had arrested him—sound familiar? Yet during his imprisonment at the Landsberg Prison, he was treated as an honored guest. There he dictated to his loyal follower Rudolf Hess chapter after chapter of the book that would become *Mein Kampf* ("My Struggle").[30]

Our salvation lies in recognizing that we must move toward implementing social and political systems that benefit all our people, or at least toward more equitably distributing those systems' risks and rewards. This will require a new vision of who we are as a people and what we want our society to achieve. From where I stand, high-quality health care for all Americans should be a right, not a privilege. But more importantly, we must plan our society going forward to reward prosocial and health-supporting practices. As my mother always said, "An ounce of prevention is worth a pound of cure." This means evaluating new technologies not by how much money they might make but by how much of a positive impact they will have on the overall health and well-being of all members of our society. With such a perspective, we never would have allowed the fast food industry to grow to its current dimensions, we never would have allowed the automobile industry to destroy public transportation in favor of freeways, and we never would have introduced PFASs into our cookware to save a few minutes of time washing up.

We are at a dark moment in our history. How we act or fail to act over the next few years will determine whether future generations will bless us for our foresight or curse us for the decisions that led to a climate catastrophe. In writing this book, I have hoped to be a blessing. It is my fervent prayer that many of you will join me in my efforts to bring about positive change.

AFTERWORD: THE LUNATICS ARE IN CHARGE OF THE ASYLUM

The bulk of this book was written in the early months of 2024. During that time, Donald Trump faced criminal indictments for hush money payments, illegally holding on to classified documents, and election interference. On February 6, 2024, a federal appeals court ruled that Trump was not immune to any charges for criminal acts committed during his presidency. However, on July 1, the Supreme Court (which had been stacked with conservative justices by Trump in his first presidency) reversed that ruling. On May 30, he was found guilty on thirty-four counts in the hush money case. On July 15, US District Judge Aileen Cannon (a Trump appointee) dismissed the classified documents case, claiming that special counsel Jack Smith's appointment violated the Constitution. After Trump won the 2024 presidential election, Smith dropped the federal election interference case. The Fulton County election interference case still stands but has been put on hold while the Georgia courts decide whether the Fulton County district attorney Fani Willis should be disqualified.[31]

Although opposed to his bid, I predicted that Donald Trump would win the 2024 presidential election despite being a convicted felon. To do so, he ran a well-organized but ideologically shallow campaign. He played on the misconceptions and fears of white Americans, a strategy employed by Republican candidates since 1968.[32] These misconceptions included that their jobs had been taken away by Blacks, Mexicans, and other immigrants and that Trump would somehow restore America's economic prowess by imposing tariffs against the nation's trade enemies. Who knew that Canada and Mexico would be on that list? For his base, "making America great again" included not just restoring economic greatness but retreating to the cultural values of the 1950s, when white supremacy went unchallenged and a marriage was between a man and a woman.

To compare Trump's first week in office to the Nazi blitzkrieg of World War II is not a stretch. His first days in office saw a dizzying array of executive orders, including one that struck down diversity, equity, and inclusion (DEI) initiatives in the federal employment and one designed to "protect American women" by declaring that gender was equivalent to biological sex. Trump's executive orders have spread confusion throughout state and federal agencies. For example, the Trump administration has forced the Food and Drug Administration to take down web pages calling for diversity in clinical trials.[33] It has also forced the Centers for Disease Control and Prevention to take down a web page providing guidance on preventing HIV transmission and preexposure prophylaxis.[34] In chapter 5, I discussed the health disparities that exist in HIV infection by socially defined race. Since these disparities exist, removing care guidelines will differentially negatively affect communities with higher infection rates. In chapter 10, I explained why diversity in clinical trials is a scientific imperative, not political correctness or woke ideology. We need more diversity in research because the more genetic diversity in clinical trials, the greater the likelihood that idiosyncratic and harmful type 2 adverse reactions will be discovered and thus prevented. No one should be opposed to the manufacture of drugs that work well for everyone. Because of the confusion caused by the Trump administration's attacks on DEI, a lecture that Andrea and I were scheduled to give on human biological diversity and medical misconceptions was canceled by the University of Kentucky College of Medicine.

Trump is also engaging in acts of vindication and vengeance. He pardoned the violent demonstrators who attacked the Capitol on January 6, 2021 (even those who had assaulted police officers), and he is currently moving to fire the FBI agents who investigated their crimes. He is attempting to remove "woke" military officers in command positions in our armed forces and replace them with officers whose loyalty to him and his agenda is without question. These actions again raise frightening parallels with the past. On January 30, 1933, Adolf Hitler was named chancellor of Germany. Within five hours, he had initiated his plan to complete the Nazification of Germany, part of which involved setting fire to the Reichstag and blaming the Communists.[35] Trump has set no physical fires (yet), but he and his party were quick to blame both the severity of the wildfires in Los Angeles County and the crash of an army helicopter into a passenger airliner on DEI.[36] It is clear from the wording of his January 2025 executive order freezing federal funding for grants and loans that Trump equates DEI with Marxism. Matthew Vaeth, the acting director of the Office of Management and Budget, stated that this was done to stop "the use of federal resources to advance Marxist equity, transgenderism, and green new deal social engineering policies."[37] J. Edgar Hoover spent much of the FBI's time and resources trying to demonstrate that the Reverend Dr. Martin Luther King Jr. was a communist. No such evidence was ever found.[38]

Trump is currently engaged in a program to gut the parts of the federal government that he feels are in opposition to his program. This includes removing longtime federal workers in agencies who work on projects related to climate change and those who conduct research in areas like women's health and gender identity issues. His targets indicate that this administration is cherry-picking its science. On one hand, it wants to spend billions of dollars to build more powerful artificial intelligence; on the other, it is attempting to dismiss or underfund issues it has no use for. Eliminating areas of research that have decades of solid evidence supporting them is like telling the American people that the earth is flat. Anthropogenic climate change is real and causing serious problems globally. There is no gender binary.

Gender is fluid and influenced by one's genetics, developmental environment, epigenetics, brain structure, hormone levels, and genitalia.

To further his plan to incapacitate historically underserved communities, Trump has targeted the Department of Education for elimination. The functions of this agency may be reorganized into others, or moneys may be given directly to the states in block grants. Should the latter happen, we should remember that the former Confederate states have a record of diverting moneys earmarked for racially subordinated groups toward funding for education for socially advantaged groups.[39] He is also making drastic cuts to the workforce of the National Science Foundation, which are being implemented via a campaign of intimidation in which federal employees are being offered the opportunity to retire and take a payout or face the threat of being laid off.[40]

As part of his plan to "make America great again," Trump has appointed individuals to cabinet positions based not on experience, knowledge of the position's charge, or competence but rather on their loyalty to him and his agenda. If Trump succeeds with this plan, it will be hard to assess the harm that will be done to racialized people, to poor people, to LGBTQ+ people, and to women across the nation. What is clear is that, should we survive this, it will take generations to undo the damage. However, of all Trump's appointees, that of Robert F. Kennedy Jr. as secretary of health and human services concerns me the most. Kennedy has no medical or scientific training but has taken an active role in opposing vaccination. His views on vaccination are well expressed in his 2022 book.[41] In short, despite the centuries of scientific research demonstrating the efficacy of vaccination to prevent the spread of infectious disease, Kennedy claims that vaccination does not work and that it is associated with the rise of autism in American children over the twentieth and twenty-first centuries. His claim is based on a series of discredited studies purporting that vaccines or their components are associated with increasing the risk of childhood autism. At present, the Centers for Disease Control and Prevention maintains its web page debunking this pseudoscience.[42] However, given the changes being made to federal government information sources, there is no way to know how long it will stay there.

In addition to supporting the debunked claim that vaccines cause autism, Kennedy also claims that the impact of vaccine-related autism is worse on African American children, particularly boys, than on children of other socially defined races.[43] He bases this claim on a study conducted by a researcher at the Children's Health Defense, an antivaccination organization on whose board of directors he used to serve. The study was retracted from the journal *Translational Neurodegeneration* because the author did not disclose his relationship to this organization.[44] However, the study should never have been published to begin with. There are several flaws in its design and statistical analysis. First, the author attempted to show a relationship between age of vaccination with the measles-mumps-rubella (MMR) vaccine and risk of autism. The children in the study came from the Atlanta metropolitan area. The cohort of the overall study was small, just 624 cases (children with autism) and 1,824 controls (children without autism). The analysis was conducted on children who received the vaccination at eighteen, twenty-four, and thirty-six months of age. For the African American sample, thirty-one months was used instead of thirty-six because of differences in body weight in the African American group compared to the total sample. There was no statistically significant difference in relative risk between the cases and controls at eighteen and twenty-four months in either the total sample or the African American sample. However, at thirty-six months, the relative risk between cases and controls (1.49) was statistically significant. This resulted from a greater risk in the males (1.69) since the increase in females was not statistically significant. The study further showed that the relative risk in African Americans was statistically significant (2.3) and stated that this was because of the increased risk in African American boys (3.36) (no statistically significantly increased risk was found for females). The study also reported that the increased risk in the total cohort resulted from the African Americans in the sample, which the author determined by removing the African American data and running the statistical analysis on the remainder of the sample. When this was done, no statistically significant differences between cases and controls were found at any age. If we take these results to their logical conclusion, we would expect the paper to state that the MMR vaccine did not harm children who were not African American.

However, the paper did not report the sample size of African Americans used in the statistical analysis that produced the reported odds ratio. This is a serious methodological flaw. Clearly, not all 624 children with autism in the study were African American. In 2014, the Atlanta metropolitan area was about 54 percent African American, but estimates of sample size don't matter if you don't report the numbers used in your analysis. Of course, the real problem here is that the study did *not* establish a causal link between MMR vaccination and risk of autism. The data from the non–African American sample was negative. So, we are once again left with a health disparity in African Americans that can be accounted for by a number of unspecified and unmeasured variables (see chapter 1). In 2020, the nationwide prevalence of autism spectrum disorder was 24.3, 26.5, 31.6, and 33.4 per 100,000 individuals for non-Hispanic white, American Indian/Alaska Native, non-Hispanic Black, and non-Hispanic Asian/Pacific Islander populations, respectively.[45] These figures demonstrate that population genetic diversity explains nothing about autism prevalence at all.

We should all be concerned that our new secretary of health and human services understands neither the relationship between human biological diversity and socially defined race nor their relevance to health disparities. We should be concerned that he thinks that immune response is determined by biological race. Of course, one could question how well the previous holders of this post understood these issues, but they were not attached to an administration that has taken an adamant position against anything that would improve DEI in biomedical research and clinical practice. As of this writing, Kennedy's confirmation was advanced to the full Senate on a 14–13 partisan vote. During the confirmation hearing, he repudiated his past antivaccine views but argued that vaccines might be hurting Blacks more than whites. However, we should remember that Supreme Court Justice Amy Coney Barrett said she would not oppose *Roe v. Wade* during her Senate confirmation, and look how that turned out. Thus, we can't know how Kennedy will behave relative to the development and deployment of vaccines.

During the revision of this conclusion, Kennedy was confirmed as the Secretary of Health and Human Services. As expected, he has already begun to sow doubt concerning the efficacy of vaccination and resurrected the pseudoscientific connection between vaccination and autism. On April 10, 2025, he claimed that the new research program that he is initiating will find the cause of the "autism epidemic" by September 2025.[46] This hubris concerning the complexity of disease causation can only be exhibited by someone who knows absolutely nothing about the nature of the scientific method. Of course, the simplest explanation for his bravado is that he has already decided what his research program is going to find: that this can all be explained by vaccination.

CONCLUSION

In chapter 5, I discussed how pathogens are constantly evolving and how the conditions of human life precondition them for successful transmission in our species. We are thus in a constant struggle to develop methods to control them. Vaccines are an essential tool in our arsenal of antimicrobials. Their efficacy may vary by individual but certainly not by socially defined race. Unfortunately, in the new regime, we will have an even harder time teaching those lessons to biomedical researchers and clinicians. We cannot allow the inmates to control the asylum much longer. The cost may be more than we can bear.

NOTES

PREFACE

1. J. L. Graves and A. Goodman, *Racism, Not Race: Answers to Frequently Asked Questions* (Columbia University Press, 2022).

INTRODUCTION: MEDICINE HAS ALWAYS
GOTTEN RACE WRONG

The epigraph is taken from R. B. Sheridan, "The Guinea Surgeons on the Middle Passage: The Provision of Medical Services in the British Slave Trade," *International Journal of African Historical Studies* 14, no. 4 (1981): 601–25.

1. P. D. Curtin, *The Atlantic Slave Trade: A Census* (University of Wisconsin Press, 1969).
2. S. M. Mustakeem, *Slavery at Sea: Terror, Sex, and Sickness in the Middle Passage* (University of Illinois Press, 2016).
3. C. S. Wilder, *Ebony and Ivy: Race, Slavery, and the Troubled History of American Universities* (Bloomsbury, 2013).
4. C. D. E. Willoughby, "Running Away from Drapetomania: Samuel A. Cartwright, Medicine, and Race in the Antebellum South," *Journal of Southern History* 84, no. 3 (2018): 571–614.
5. J. S. Haller, "The Negro and the Southern Physician: A Study of Medical and Racial Attitudes 1800–1860, *Medical History* 16 (1972): 238–53.
6. Abrahams and Parsons, 1996. P. W. Abrahams and J. A. Parsons, "Geophagy in the Tropics: A Literature Review," *Geographical Journal* 162, no. 1 (1996): 63–72.
7. A. Derickson, "'A Widespread Superstition': The Purported Invulnerability of Workers of Color to Occupational Heat Stress," *American Journal of Public Health* 109, no. 10 (2019): 1329–35.

8. J. L. Graves, *The Emperor's New Clothes: Biological Theories of Race at the Millennium* (Rutgers University Press, 2005).

9. S. J. Gould, *The Mismeasure of Man* (Norton, 1981).

10. Willoughby, "Running Away."

11. D. C. Owens and S. M. Fett, "Black Maternal and Infant Health: Historical Legacies of Slavery," *American Journal of Public Health* 109, no. 10 (2019): 1342–45.

12. J. Downs, *Sick from Freedom: African American Illness and Suffering During the Civil War and Reconstruction* (Oxford University Press, 2012).

13. K. M. Stampp, *The Era of Reconstruction: 1865–1877* (Vintage, 1967).

14. A. Planas, "New Florida Standards Teach Students That Some Black People Benefited From Slavery Because It Taught Useful Skills, NBC News, July 20, 2023; https://www.nbcnews.com/news/us-news/new-florida-standards-teach-black-people-benefited-slavery-taught-usef-rcna95418.

15. Graves, *The Emperor's New Clothes*, 177–78.

16. F. L. Hoffman, *The Race Traits and Tendencies of the American Negro* (Andrus & Church, 1896).

17. See, for example, H. R. Ramsey, "The Southern Negro," *Philadelphia Medical Surgery Journal* (1852–53): 293–99; S. L. Grier, "The Negro and His Diseases," *New Orleans Medical Surgery Journal* 9 (1852–53): 752–63; F. Tipton, "The Negro Problem from a Medical Standpoint," *New York Medical Journal* 43 (1886): 570; S. Harris, "The Future of the Negro from the Standpoint of the Southern Physician," *Alabama Medical Journal* 14 (1902): 60.

18. Graves, *The Emperor's New Clothes*, chap. 8.

19. A. Chase, *The Legacy of Malthus: The Social Costs of the New Scientific Racism* (University of Illinois Press, 1980).

20. D. C. Ewbank, "History of Black Mortality and Health Before 1940," *Milbank Quarterly* 65, no. S1 (1987): 100–128.

21. J. L. Graves, "Looking at the World Through 'Race' Colored Glasses: The Influence of Ascertainment Bias on Biomedical Research and Practice," in *Mapping "Race": A Critical Reader on Health Disparities Research*, ed. Laura Gomez and Nancy Lopez (Rutgers University Press, 2013).

22. J. L. Graves, *The Race Myth: Why We Pretend Race Exists in America* (Dutton, 2005).

23. C. Caraballo et al., "Excess Mortality and Years of Potential Life Lost Among the Black Population in the US, 1999–2020," *Journal of the American Medical Association* 329, no. 19 (2023):1662–70; A. Johnson, "Black Communities Endured Wave of Excess Deaths in Past 2 Decades, Studies Find: The Loss of Life Came at a Staggering Cost, Medically and Economically," *Washington Post*, May 16, 2023, https://www.washingtonpost.com/health/2023/05/16/black-communities-excess-deaths/.

24. S. K. Singh and K. Rajoria, "Medical Leech Therapy in Ayurveda and Biomedicine—A Review," *Journal of Ayurveda and Integrative Medicine* 11, no. 4 (2019): 554–64.

25. J. M. Barry, *The Great Influenza: The Story of the Deadliest Pandemic in History* (Penguin, 2018).

26. T. Keel, *Divine Variations: How Christian Thought Became Racial Science* (Stanford University Press, 2019).

27. A. Montagu, *Man's Most Dangerous Myth: The Fallacy of Race* (Columbia University Press, 1942).

28. R. J. Lifton, *The Nazi Doctors: Medical Killing and the Psychology of Genocide*, 2nd ed. (Basic Books, 2017).

29. T. A. Guglielmo, "'Red Cross, Double Cross': Race and America's World War II–Era Blood Donor Service," *Journal of American History* 97, no. 1 (2010): 63–90.
30. J. L. Graves, "Human Biological Variation and the 'Normal,'" *American Journal of Human Biology* 33, no. 5 (2021) e23658; R. Neese and G. C. Williams, *Why We Get Sick: The New Science of Darwinian Medicine* (Vintage, 1994); J. L. Graves, "Evolutionary Versus Racial Medicine: Why It Matters," in *Race and the Genetic Revolution: Science, Myth and Culture*, ed. S. Krimsky and K. Sloan (Columbia University Press, 2011), 142–70.
31. D. R. Dodds, "Antibiotic Resistance: A Current Epilogue," *Biochemical Pharmacology* 134 (2017): 139–46.
32. J. L. Graves et al., "Evolutionary Science as a Method to Facilitate Higher Level Thinking and Reasoning in Medical Training," *Evolution, Medicine, & Public Health* 1 (2016): 358–68; S. Stearns and R. Medzhitov, *Evolutionary Medicine* (Sinauer, 2016).
33. B. M. Donovan, "Putting Humanity Back Into the Teaching of Human Biology," *Studies in History and Philosophy of Biological and Biomedical Sciences* 52 (2015): 65–75; Graves et al., "Evolutionary Science."
34. P. I. Henry et al., "Embedded Racism: Inequitable Niche Construction as a Neglected Evolutionary Process Affecting Health," *Evolution, Medicine, & Public Health* 11, no. 1 (2023): 112–125. For more on the advancement of the importance of evolutionary biology beginning in the 1990s, see R. Nesse and G. C. Williams, *Why We Get Sick: The New Science of Darwinian Medicine* (Vintage, 1994).

1. RACIAL INJUSTICE CAUSES HEALTH INJUSTICE

1. A. M. Petro, *After the Wrath of God: AIDS, Sexuality, and American Religion* (Oxford University Press, 2015).
2. B. H. Hahn et al., "AIDS as a Zoonosis: Scientific and Public Health Implications," *Science* 287, no. 5453 (2000): 607–14; J.-C. Plantier et al., "A New Human Immunodeficiency Virus Derived from Gorillas," *Nature Medicine* 15, no. 8 (2009): 871–2.
3. B. Korber et al., "Timing the Ancestor of the HIV-1 Pandemic Strains," *Science* 288, no. 5472 (2000): 1789–96.
4. M. Worobey et al., "Direct Evidence of Extensive Diversity of HIV-1 in Kinshasa by 1960," *Nature* 455, no. 7213 (2008): 661–64.
5. D. Singh and S. V. Yi, "On the Origin and Evolution of SARS-CoV-2," *Experimental & Molecular Medicine* 53, no. 4 (2021): 537–47.
6. Y. Araf et al., "Omicron Variant of SARS-CoV-2: Genomics, Transmissibility, and Responses to Current COVID-19 Vaccines," *Journal of Medical Virology* 94, no. 5 (2022): 1825–32.
7. UNAIDS, Global Fact Sheet: World AIDS Day 2012, https://www.unaids.org/sites/default/files/media_asset/JC2434_WorldAIDSday_results_en_1.pdf.
8. M. Hunter, "Beyond the Male-Migrant: South Africa's Long History of Health Geography," *Health and Place* 16 (2016): 25–33.
9. W. C. Chirwa, "Aliens and AIDS in Southern Africa: The Malawi-South Africa Debate," *African Affairs* 97 (1998): 53–79; G. J. Bell et al., "Race, Place, and HIV: The Legacies of Apartheid and Racist Policy in South Africa," *Social Science and Medicine* 296 (2022): 114755.
10. A. Mhungu et al., "Adolescent Girls and Young Women's Experiences of Living with HIV in the Context of Patriarchal Culture in Sub-Saharan Africa: A Scoping Review," *AIDS and Behavior* 27 (2023): 1365–79.

11. G. Foster and J. Williamson. "A Review of the Current Literature of the Impact of HIV/AIDS on Children in Sub-Saharan Africa," *AIDS* 14, no. S3 (2000): S275–84.

12. V. Kumar et al., *Robbins & Kumar Basic Pathology*, 11th ed. (Elsevier, 2023).

13. A. Li et al., "Race in the Reading: A Study of Problematic Uses of Race and Ethnicity in a Prominent Pediatrics Textbook," *Academic Medicine* 97, no. 10 (2022): 1521–27.

14. J. L. Graves and A. Goodman. *Racism, Not Race: Answers to Frequently Asked Questions* (Columbia University Press), 82–112.

15. Johns Hopkins University, OMIM: An Online Catalog of Human Genes and Genetic Disorders, https://www.omim.org/.

16. J. C. Herron and S. Freeman, *Evolutionary Analysis*, 5th ed. (Pearson, 2015).

17. R. Lewis, *Human Genetics: Concepts and Applications*, 5th ed. (McGraw-Hill, 2003).

18. P. Hardelid et al., "The Birth Prevalence of PKU in Populations of European, South Asian and Sub-Saharan African Ancestry Living in South East England," *Annals of Human Genetics* 72, pt. 1 (2008): 65–71.

19. A. M. Paquette et al., "The Evolutionary Origins of Southeast Asian Ovalocytosis," *Infection, Genetics and Evolution* 34 (2015): 153–59.

20. S. Michalakis et al., "Achromatopsia: Genetics and Gene Therapy," *Molecular Diagnosis & Therapy* 26, no. 1 (2022): 51–59.

21. T. W. Simon, "Defining Genocide," *Wisconsin International Law Journal* 15 (1996): 243–56.

22. A Kwan et al., "Successful Newborn Screening for SCID in the Navajo Nation," *Clinical Immunology* 158, no. 1 (2015): 29–34.

23. "The Long Walk," Smithsonian National Museum of the American Indian, accessed October 15, 2021, https://americanindian.si.edu/nk360/navajo/long-walk/long-walk.cshtml.

24. R. Dunbar-Ortiz, *An Indigenous People's History of the United States*, (Beacon, 2014).

25. Li et al., "A Founder Mutation in Artemis, an SNM1-like Protein, Causes SCID in Athabascan-Speaking Native Americans," *Journal of Immunology* 168 (2002): 6323–29.

26. P. W. Hedrick, "Population Genetics of Malaria Resistance in Humans," *Heredity* 107 (2011): 283–304; P. W. Hedrick, "Resistance to Malaria in Humans: The Impact of Strong, Recent Selection," *Malaria Journal* 11 (2012): 349.

27. T. L. Savitt, "Black Health on the Plantation: Owners, the Enslaved, and Physicians," *OAH Magazine of History* 19, no. 5 (2005): 14–16.

28. J. Abbasi, "Taking a Closer Look at COVID-19, Health Inequities, and Racism," *JAMA* 324 (2020): 427–29.

29. National Center for Health Statistics, "National Vital Statistics Reports," Centers for Disease Control and Prevention, 2019 (last reviewed September 29, 2023), https://www.cdc.gov/nchs/products/nvsr.htm.

30. K. Churchwell, et al., "Call to Action: Structural Racism as a Fundamental Driver of Health Disparities: A Presidential Advisory from the American Heart Association," *Circulation* 142 (2020): e454–68.

31. M. E. Pepin et al., "Racial and Socioeconomic Disparity Associates with Differences in Cardiac DNA Methylation Among Men with End-Stage Heart Failure," *American Journal of Physiology, Heart and Circulatory Physiology* 320 (2021): H2066–79.

32. S. Stearns and R. Medzhitov, *Evolutionary Medicine* (Sinauer, 2016).

33. T. I. Demcollari et al., "Phenotypic Plasticity in the Pancreas: New Triggers, New Players," *Current Opinion in Cell Biology* 49 (2017): 38–46.

34. M. A. Fleming et al., "Food Insecurity and Obesity in US Adolescents: A Population-Based Analysis," *Childhood Obesity* 17, no. 2 (2021): 110–15.

35. P. Medawar, *An Unsolved Problem in Biology* (H. K. Lewis), 1952; G. C. Williams, "Pleiotropy, Natural Selection, and the Evolution of Senescence," *Evolution* 11 (1957) 398–411.

36. M. K. Burke et al., "Genome-Wide Analysis of a Long-Term Evolution Experiment with *Drosophila.*" *Nature* 467, no. 7315 (2010): 587–90.

37. J. L. Graves et al., "Genomics of Parallel Experimental Evolution *in Drosophila,*" *Molecular Biology and Evolution* 34, no. 4 (2017): 831–42.

38. "Huntington Disease," OMIM.org, June 4, 1985 (last updated December 1, 2022), https://www.omim.org/entry/143100?search=%22huntington%20chorea%22&highlight =%22huntington%20chorea%22#264; J. Palo et al., "Low Prevalence of Huntington's Disease in Finland," *Lancet* 330 (1987): 805–806.

39. J. L. Graves. "General Theories of Aging, Unification and Synthesis," in *Principles of Neural Aging*, ed. Sergio F. Dani, Akira Hori, and Gerhard F. Walter (Elsevier, 1997), 35–55.

40. R. Nesse, *Good Reasons for Bad Feelings: Insights from the Frontiers of Evolutionary Psychiatry* (Dutton, 2019).

41. Kumar et al., *Robbins & Kumar.*

42. H. K. Hughes et al., "Pediatric Asthma Health Disparities: Race, Hardship, Housing, and Asthma in a National Survey," *Academic Pediatrics* 17, no. 2 (2017): 127–34.

43. W. E. B. Du Bois, *The Philadelphia Negro: A Social Study* (University of Pennsylvania Press, 1899).

44. E. Rosenbaum, "Racial/Ethnic Differences in Home Ownership and Housing Quality, 1991," *Social Problems* 43, no. 4 (1996): 403–26; G. G. Shelton et al., "Profiles and Perspectives of Housing Quality of Blacks in Selected Southern Metropolitan Cities," *Housing and Society* 23, no. 2 (1996): 84–110.

45. M. Neal et al., *Implications of Housing Conditions for Racial Wealth and Health Disparities* (Urban Institute, 2024), https://www.urban.org/sites/default/files/2024-01 /Implications%20of%20Housing%20Conditions%20for%20Racial%20Wealth%20 and%20Health%20Disparities_0.pdf.

46. A. Nardone et al., "Associations Between Historical Residential Redlining and Current Age-Adjusted Rates of Emergency Department Visits Due to Asthma Across Eight Cities in California: An Ecological Study," *Lancet Planetary Health* 4, no. 1 (2020): e24–31.

47. X. Xu, et al., "A Genomewide Search for Quantitative-Trait Loci Underlying Asthma," *American Journal of Human Genetics* 69, no. 6 (2001): 1271–77.

48. A.M. Levin et al., "Nocturnal Asthma and the Importance of Race/Ethnicity and Genetic Ancestry," *American Journal of Respiratory and Critical Care Medicine* 190, no. 3 (2014): 266–73.

49. B. A. Martin-Giacalone et al., "Prevalence and Descriptive Epidemiology of Turner Syndrome in the United States, 2000–2017: A Report from the National Birth Defects Prevention Network," *American Journal of Medical Genetics A* 191, no. 5 (2023): 1339–49.

50. P.-E. Bouet et al., "Fertility and Pregnancy in Turner Syndrome," *Journal of Obstetrics and Gynaecology Canada* 38, no. 8 (2016): 712–18.

51. R. Wiersma, "True Hermaphroditism in Southern Africa: The Clinical Picture," *Pediatric Surgery International* 20 (2004): 363–68.

52. Stearns and Medzhitov, *Evolutionary Medicine.*

53. V. Steinthorsdottir et al., "Genetic Predisposition to Hypertension Is Associated with Preeclampsia in European and Central Asian Women," *Nature Communications* 11 (2020): 5976.

54. C. Giurgescu et al., "Relationships Among Psychosocial Factors, Biomarkers, Pre-eclampsia, and Preterm Birth in African American Women: A Pilot," *Applied Nursing Research* 28 (2015): e1–6.

55. C. Giurgescu and D. P. Misra, "Psychosocial Factors and Preterm Birth Among Black Mothers and Fathers," *MCN: The American Journal of Maternal/Child Nursing* 43 (2018): 245–51.

56. W. A. Grobman et al., "Racial Disparities in Adverse Pregnancy Outcomes and Psychosocial Stress," *Obstetrics & Gynecology* 131, no. 2 (2018): 328–35.

57. J. L. Graves, *The Emperor's New Clothes: Biological Theories of Race at the Millennium* (Rutgers University Press, 2001).

58. P. I. Henry, M. R. Spence Beaulieu, A. Bradford, and J. L. Graves. "Embedded Racism: Inequitable Niche Construction as a Neglected Evolutionary Process Affecting Health," *Evolution, Medicine, and Public Health* 11, no. 1 (2023):112–25.

2. DON'T BLAME IT ON PANDORA

1. Genesis 3:16–19 (New International Bible).

2. U. Beier, ed., *The Origin of Life & Death: African Creation Myths* (East African, 1966).

3. S. Lindeburg, *Food and Western Disease: Health and Nutrition from an Evolutionary Perspective* (Wiley-Blackwell), 2010.

4. J. L. Graves, "Out of Africa: Where Faith, Race, and Science Collide," in *Critical Approaches to Science and Religion*, ed. M. P. Sheldon, A. Ragab, and T. Keel (Columbia University Press, 2023).

5. J. M. Barry, *The Great Influenza: The Story of the Deadliest Pandemic in History* (Penguin, 2018); A. R. Butler and J. L. Hogg, "Exploring Scotland's Influenza Pandemic of 1918–19: Lest We Forget," *Journal of the Royal College of Physicians of Edinburgh* 37, no. 4 (2007): 362–66.

6. L. Li et al., "Recurrent Gene Flow Between Neanderthals and Modern Humans Over the Past 200,000 Years," *Science* 385, no. 6705 (2024): eadi1768.

7. J. L. Graves, *A Voice in the Wilderness: A Pioneering Biologist Explains How Evolution Can Help Us Solve Our Biggest Problems* (Basic Books, 2022).

8. S. Ellis et al., "Postreproductive Lifespans Are Rare in Mammals," *Ecology and Evolution* 8, no. 5 (2018): 2482–94.

9. G. C. Williams, "Pleiotropy, Natural Selection, and the Evolution of Senescence," *Evolution* 11 (1957): 398–411.

10. Graves, *A Voice in the Wilderness*, 81–97.

11. M. R. Rose, "Laboratory Evolution of Postponed Senescence in *Drosophila melanogaster*," *Evolution* 38, no. 5 (1984): 1004–10; L. S. Luckinbill et al., "Selection for Delayed Senescence in *Drosophila melanogaster*," *Evolution* 38, no. 5 (1984): 996–1003.

12. J. L. Graves et al., "Desiccation, Flight, Glycogen and Postponed Senescence in *Drosophila melanogaster*," *Physiological Zoology* 65, no. 2 (1992): 268–86.

13. J. R. Speakman and S. E. Mitchell, "Caloric Restriction," *Molecular Aspects of Medicine*, 32, no. 3 (2011): 159–221.

14. J. L. Graves, "The Costs of Reproduction and Dietary Restriction in Mammals," *Growth, Development, and Aging* 57, no. 4 (1993): 233–49.

15. L. Harries et al., "The Biology of Ageing and the Omics Revolution," *Biogerontology* 19, no. 6 (2018): 435–36.

16. J. E. Fleming et al., "Two-Dimensional Protein Analysis of Postponed Aging in *Drosophila*," in *Methuselah Flies: A Case Study in the Evolution of Aging*, ed. M. R. Rose, H. B. Passananti, and M. Matos (World Scientific, 2004), 205–20.

17. D. Graur, *Molecular and Genome Evolution* (Sinauer, 2016).

18. J. L. Graves et al., "Genomics of Parallel Experimental Evolution in *Drosophila*," *Molecular Biology and Evolution* 34, no. 4 (2017): 831–42.

19. K. P. Murphy et al., *Janeway's Immunobiology* (Garland Science, 2008).

20. H. M. Dönertaş et al., "Common Genetic Associations Between Age-Related Diseases," *Nature Aging* 1, no. 4 (2021): 400–412. A description of the individuals whose data is found in the UK Biobank can be found at https://www.ukbiobank.ac.uk/.

21. E. Long and J. Zhang, "Evidence for the Role of Selection for Reproductively Advantageous Alleles in Human Aging," *Science Advances* 9, no. 49 (2023): eadh4990.

22. S. G. Byars and K. Voskarides, "Antagonistic Pleiotropy in Human Disease," *Journal of Molecular Evolution* 88, no. 1 (2020): 12–25.

23. S. Stearns and R. Medzhitov, *Evolutionary Medicine* (Sinauer, 2016), 28.

24. K. R. Smith et al., "Effects of *BRCA1* and *BRCA2* Mutations on Female Fertility," *Proceedings of the Royal Society B* 279, no. 1732 (2012): 1389–95.

25. K. M. Im et al., "Haplotype Structure in Ashkenazi Jewish *BRCA1* and *BRCA2* Mutation Carriers," *Human Genetics* 130, no. 5 (2011): 685–99.

26. D. L. Bodian et al., "Germline Variation in Cancer-Susceptibility Genes in a Healthy, Ancestrally Diverse Cohort: Implications for Individual Genome Sequencing," *PLoS One* 9, no. 4 (2014): e94554.

27. J. L. Graves and A. Goodman, *Racism, Not Race: Answers to Frequently Asked Questions* (Columbia University Press, 2022).

28. T. Dobzhansky, "Nothing Makes Sense Save in the Light of Evolution," *American Biology Teacher* 35, no. 3 (1973): 125–29.

29. R. M. Nesse and G. C. Williams, *Why We Get Sick: The New Science of Darwinian Medicine* (Norton, 1994).

30. J. L. Graves, "Why Do We Age and Can We Fix It?," *Culturico*, February 3, 2023, https://culturico.com/2023/02/03/why-do-we-age-and-can-we-fix-it/.

3. THERE IS NO SLAVERY GENE:
DEBUNKING THE MYTHS OF HYPERTENSION

1. J. L. Graves, *The Emperor's New Clothes: Biological Theories of Race at the Millennium* (Rutgers University Press, 2005).

2. C. D. Fryar et al., "Hypertension Prevalence and Control Among Adults: United States, 2015–2016," *NCHS Data Brief* no. 289 (2017): 1–8.

3. S. F. Mohamed et al., "Prevalence of Uncontrolled Hypertension in People with Comorbidities in Sub-Saharan Africa: A Systematic Review and Meta-analysis," *BMJ Open* 11, no. 12 (2021): e045880.

4. A. D. Kaze, et al., "Prevalence of Hypertension in Older People in Africa: A Systematic Review and Meta-analysis," *Journal of Hypertension* 35, no. 7 (2017): 1345–52.

5. F. Ataklte et al., "Burden of Undiagnosed Hypertension in Sub-Saharan Africa: A Systematic Review and Meta-analysis," *Hypertension* 65, no. 2 (2015): 291–98.

6. V. Kumar et al., *Robbins & Kumar Basic Pathology*, 10th ed. (Elsevier, 2019).

7. P. Song et al., "Global Prevalence of Hypertension in Children: A Systematic Review and Meta-analysis," *JAMA Pediatrics* 173, no. 12 (2019): 1154–63.

8. J. J. Carvalho et a., "Blood Pressure in Four Remote Populations in the INTERSALT Study," *Hypertension* 14, no. 3 (1989): 238–46.

9. D. Adeloye et al., "An Estimate of the Prevalence of Hypertension in Nigeria: A Systematic Review and Meta-analysis," *Journal of Hypertension* 33, no. 3 (2015): 230–42.

10. S. J. Micheletti et al., "Genetic Consequences of the Transatlantic Slave Trade in the Americas," *American Journal of Human Genetics* 107, no. 2 (2020): 265–77.

11. M. Bijani et al., "Investigating the Prevalence of Hypertension and Its Associated Risk Factors in a Population-Based Study: Fasa PERSIAN COHORT Data," *BMC Cardiovascular Disorders* 20, no. 1 (2020): 503.

12. M. T. Nguyen and D. H. Rehkopf, "Prevalence of Chronic Disease and Their Risk Factors Among Iranian, Ukrainian, Vietnamese Refugees in California, 2002–2011," *Journal of Immigrant and Minority Health* 18, no. 6 (2016): 1274–83.

13. V. Kumar et al., *Robbins & Kumar Basic Pathology*, 11th ed. (Elsevier, 2023).

14. K. Bryc et al., "The Genetic Ancestry of African Americans, Latinos, and European Americans Across the United States," *American Journal of Human Genetics* 96, no. 1 (2015): 37–53.

15. H. Kaur, et al., "Replication of European Hypertension Associations in a Case-Control Study of 9,534 African Americans," *PLoS One* 16, no. 11 (2021): e0259962.

16. J. S. Kaufman and S. A. Hall, "The Slavery Hypertension Hypothesis: Dissemination and Appeal of a Modern Race Theory," *Epidemiology* 14, no. 1 (2003): 111–18.

17. Graves, *The Emperor's New Clothes.*

18. P. Rust and C. Ekmekcioglu, "Impact of Salt Intake on the Pathogenesis and Treatment of Hypertension," *Advances in Experimental Medicine and Biology* 956 (2017): 61–84.

19. J. C. K. Wells, *The Metabolic Ghetto: An Evolutionary Perspective on Nutrition, Power Relations, and Chronic Disease* (Cambridge University Press, 2016).

20. M. O'Hearn et al., "Trends and Disparities in Cardiometabolic Health Among U.S. Adults, 1999–2018," *Journal of the American College of Cardiology* 80, no. 2 (2022): 138–51.

21. O'Hearn et al., "Trends and Disparities."

22. J. B. Meigs, "The Genetic Epidemiology of Type 2 Diabetes: Opportunities for Health Translation," *Current Diabetes Reports* 19, no. 8 (2019): 62.

23. L. K. Billings and J. C. Florez, "The Genetics of Type 2 Diabetes: What Have We Learned from GWAS?," *Annals of the New York Academy of Sciences* 1212 (2010): 59–77.

24. J. L. Vassy et al., "Polygenic Type 2 Diabetes Prediction at the Limit of Common Variant Detection," *Diabetes* 63, no. 6 (2014): 2172–82.

25. S. Dawson, *The Lost Colony and Hatteras Island* (History, 2020).

26. J. L. Graves and A. Goodman, *Racism, Not Race: Answers to Frequently Asked Questions* (Columbia University Press, 2022), chap. 4; R. Dunbar-Ortiz R, *An Indigenous People's History of the United States* (Beacon, 2014).

27. P. Ivey et al., "Embedded Racism: Inequitable Niche Construction as a Neglected Evolutionary Process Affecting Health," *Evolution, Medicine, and Public Health* 11, no. 1 (2023): 112–25.

28. N. Snyder-Mackler et al., "Social Determinants of Health and Survival in Humans and Other Animals," *Science* 368, no. 6493 (2020): eaax9553.

29. M. L. Sells et al., "Excess Burden of Poverty and Hypertension, by Race and Ethnicity, on the Prevalence of Cardiovascular Disease," *Preventing Chronic Disease* 20 (2023): E109; L. Malan and N. T. Malan, "Emotional Stress as a Risk for Hypertension

in Sub-Saharan Africans: Are We Ignoring the Odds?," *Advances in Experimental Medicine and Biology* 956 (2017): 497–510; J. A. Hanson and M. R. Huecker, "Sleep Deprivation," in *StatPearls* (Stat Pearls, 2023), https://www.ncbi.nlm.nih.gov/books /NBK547676/; C. M. Dolezsar et al., "Perceived Racial Discrimination and Hypertension: A Comprehensive Systematic Review," *Health Psychology* 33, no. 1 (2014): 20–34; Z. Huang, "Association Between Blood Lead Level with High Blood Pressure in US (NHANES 1999–2018)," *Frontiers in Public Health* 10 (2022): 836357; C. Koh et al., "Socioeconomic Disparities in Hypertension by Levels of Green Space Availability: A Cross-Sectional Study in Philadelphia, PA," *International Journal of Environmental Research and Public Health* 19, no. 4 (2022): 2037.

30. R. D. Bullard et al., *Toxic Wastes and Race at Twenty, 1987–2007: A Report Prepared for the United Church of Christ Justice & Witness Ministries* (United Church of Christ, 2007), https://www.ucc.org/wp-content/uploads/2021/03/toxic-wastes-and-race-at-twenty -1987-2007.pdf.

31. Graves and Goodman, *Racism, Not Race.*

4. RACE AND THE MICROBIOME

1. D. Dykhuizen, "Species Numbers in Bacteria," *Proceedings of the California Academy of Sciences* 56, no. 6 Suppl. 1 (2005): 62–71.

2. M. Woolhouse et al., "Human Viruses: Discovery and Emergence," *Philosophical Transactions of the Royal Society B* 367, no. 1604 (2012): 2864–71.

3. L. K. Ursell et al., "Defining the Human Microbiome," *Nutrition Reviews* 70, no. S1 (2012): S38–44.

4. I. A. Hatton et al., "The Human Cell Count and Size Distribution," *Proceedings of the National Academy of Sciences of the United States of America* 120, no. 39 (2023): e2303077120.

5. J. E. Wilkinson et al., "A Framework for Microbiome Science in Public Health," *Nature Medicine* 27, no. 5 (2021): 766–74.

6. E. R. Davenport et al., "The Human Microbiome in Evolution," *BMC Biology* 15, no. 1 (2017): 127.

7. N. A. Lerminiaux and A. D. S. Cameron, "Horizontal Transfer of Antibiotic Resistance Genes in Clinical Environments," *Canadian Journal of Microbiology* 65, no. 1 (2019): 34–44.

8. J. Lloyd-Price et al., "The Healthy Human Microbiome," *Genome Medicine* 8, no. 1 (2016): 51.

9. P. Vangay et al., "US Immigration Westernizes the Human Gut Microbiome," *Cell* 175, no. 4 (2018): 962–72.

10. M. H. Y. Leung et al., "Insights into the Pan-microbiome: Skin Microbial Communities of Chinese Individuals Differ from Other Racial Groups," *Scientific Reports* 5 (2015): 11845; M. H. Y. Leung et al., "Erratum: Insights into the Pan-microbiome: Skin Microbial Communities of Chinese Individuals Differ from Other Racial Groups," *Scientific Reports* 6 (2016): 21355.

11. M. Deschasaux et al., "Depicting the Composition of Gut Microbiota in a Population with Varied Ethnic Origins but Shared Geography," *Nature Medicine* 24 (2018): 1526–31.

12. L. C. Conteville and A. C. P. Vicente, "Skin Exposure to Sunlight: A Factor Modulating the Human Gut Microbiome Composition," *Gut Microbes* 11, no. 5 (2020): 1135–38.

13. A. W. Brooks et al., "Gut Microbiota Diversity Across Ethnicities in the United States," *PLoS Biology* 16, no. 12 (2018): e2006842.
14. K. Bryc et al., "The Genetic Ancestry of African Americans, Latinos, and European Americans Across the United States," *American Journal of Human Genetics* 96, no. 1 (2015): 37–53.
15. T. L. Carson et al., "Associations Between Race, Perceived Psychological Stress, and the Gut Microbiota in a Sample of Generally Healthy Black and White Women: A Pilot Study on the Role of Race and Perceived Psychological Stress," *Psychosomatic Medicine* 80, no. 7 (2018): 640–48.
16. L. Farhana et al., "Gut Microbiome Profiling and Colorectal Cancer in African Americans and Caucasian Americans," *World Journal of Gastrointestinal Pathophysiology* 9, no. 2 (2018): 47–58.
17. A. Tomova et al., "The Effects of Vegetarian and Vegan Diets on Gut Microbiota. *Frontiers in Nutrition* 6 (2019): 47.
18. I. Martínez I et al., "Resistant Starches Types 2 and 4 Have Differential Effects on the Composition of the Fecal Microbiota in Human Subjects," *PLoS One* 5, no. 11 (2010): e15046.
19. Conteville and Vincente, "Skin Exposure to Sunlight."
20. M. Sogin, "Trying to Makes Sense of the Microbial Census," in *Microbes and Evolution: The World That Darwin Never Saw*, ed. R. Kolter and S. Maloy (ASM, 2012):30–36.
21. Y. Zha et al., "Microbial Dark Matter: From Discovery to Applications," *Genomics Proteomics Bioinformatics* 20, no. 5 (2022): 867–81.
22. J. L. Graves et al., "Inequality in Science and the Case for a New Agenda," *Proceedings of the National Academy of Sciences of the United States of America* 119, no. 10 (2022): e2117831119; E. A. Cech, "The Intersectional Privilege of White Able-Bodied Heterosexual Men in STEM," *Science Advances* 8, no. 24 (2022): eabo1558.
23. J. L. Graves, "Human Biological Variation and the 'Normal,'" *American Journal of Human Biology* 33, no. 5 (2021): e23658; National Academies of Sciences, Engineering, and Medicine, *Using Population Descriptors in Genetics and Genomics Research: A New Framework for an Evolving Field* (National Academies Press, 2023).
24. D. S. Falconer and T. Mackay, *Introduction to Quantitative Genetics*, 4th ed. (Longman, 1996).
25. J. L. Graves and A. Goodman, *Racism, Not Race: Answers to Frequently Asked Questions* (Columbia University Press, 2022), chaps. 4 and 5.
26. A. Kurilshikov et al., "Large-scale Association Analyses Identify Host Factors Influencing Human Gut Microbiome Composition," *Nature Genetics* 53, no. 2 (2021):156–65.
27. E. A. Mayer et al., "The Gut–Brain Axis," *Annual Review of Medicine* 73 (2022): 439–53.
28. Graves et al., "Inequality in Science."
29. K. J. Royston et al., "Race, the Microbiome and Colorectal Cancer," *World Journal of Gastrointestinal Oncology* 11, no. 10 (2019): 773–87; A. S. Wilson et al., "Diet and the Human Gut Microbiome: An International Review," *Digestive Diseases and Sciences* 65, no. 3 (2022): 723–40; K. R. Amato et al., "The Human Gut Microbiome and health Inequities," *Proceedings of the National Academy of Sciences of the United States of America* 118, no. 25 (2021): e2017947118; S. Sun et al., "Race, the Vaginal Microbiome, and Spontaneous Preterm Birth," *mSystems* 7, no. 3 (2022): e0001722.
30. D. L. Merrifield et al., "Ingestion of Metal-Nanoparticle Contaminated Food Disrupts Endogenous Microbiota in Zebrafish (*Danio rerio*)," *Environmental Pollution* 174 (2013): 157–63.

31. S. Assefa and G. Köhler, "Intestinal Microbiome and Metal Toxicity," *Current Opinion in Toxicology* 19 (2020): 21–27.
32. M. Hanna-Attisha et al., "Elevated Blood Lead Levels in Children Associated with the Flint Drinking Water Crisis: A Spatial Analysis of Risk and Public Health Response," *American Journal of Public Health* 106, no. 2 (2016): 283–90.
33. M. Hanna-Attisha et al., "Elevated Blood Lead Levels."

5. INFECTIOUS DISEASE STRIKES UNEVENLY: THE POOR DIE MORE

1. J. L. Graves, *Principles and Applications of Antimicrobial Nanomaterials* (Elsevier, 2021), chap. 11.
2. D. Dykhuizen, "Species Numbers in Bacteria," *Proceedings of the California Academy of Sciences* 56, no. 6 Suppl. 1 (2005): 62–71; K. J. Locey and J. T. Lennon, "Scaling Laws Predict Global Microbial Diversity," *Proceedings of the National Academy of Sciences of the United States of America* 113, no. 21 (2016): 5970–75.
3. A. Bartlett et al., "A Comprehensive List of Bacterial Pathogens Infecting Humans," *Microbiology (Reading)* 168, no. 12 (2022); M. Woolhouse et al., "Human Viruses: Discovery and Emergence," *Philosophical Transactions of the Royal Society of London, Series B, Biological Sciences* 367, no. 1604 (2012): 2864–71.
4. M. D. Cooper and M. N. Alder, "The Evolution of Adaptive Immune Systems," *Cell* 124, no. 4 (2006): 815–22.
5. G. Sorci G and B. Faivre, "Age-Dependent Virulence of Human Pathogens," *PLoS Pathogens* 18, no. 9 (2022): e1010866.
6. Roland S. Martin, "Gen. Lloyd Austin (Ret) Talks COVID-19; States Announce Shutdowns; Protecting Your $ During Outbreak," *Roland Martin Unfiltered Daily Digital Show*, interview with Joseph L. Graves Jr., posted March 20, 2020, YouTube, https://youtu.be/rtRI5hLJ7hc.
7. A. Nguyen et al., "Human Leukocyte Antigen Susceptibility Map for Severe Acute Respiratory Syndrome Coronavirus 2," *Journal of Virology* 94, no. 13 (2020): e00510–20.
8. J. L. Graves, "Their Money, Our Lives," *Science for the People*, August 23, 2020, https://magazine.scienceforthepeople.org/online/covid-19-coronanvirus-wealth-race-public-health/.
9. R. A. Oppel et al., "The Fullest Look Yet at the Racial Inequality of Coronavirus," *New York Times*, July 5, 2020, https://www.nytimes.com/interactive/2020/07/05/us/coronavirus-latinos-african-americans-cdc-data.html?action=click&module=RelatedLinks&pgtype=Article.
10. M. Li and F. Yuan, "Historical Redlining and Resident Exposure to COVID-19: A Study of New York City," *Race and Social Problems* 14, no. 2 (2022): 85–100.
11. "COVID-19 Among Workers in Meat and Poultry Processing Facilities—19 States, April 2020," *Morbidity and Mortality Weekly Report*, May 8, 2020, https://www.cdc.gov/mmwr/volumes/69/wr/mm6918e3.htm?s_cid=mm6918e3_w.
12. K. Kindy et al., "The Trump Administration Approved Faster Line Speeds at Chicken Plants. Those Facilities Are More Likely to Have COVID-19 Cases," *Washington Post*, January 3, 2021, https://www.washingtonpost.com/politics/trump-chicken-covid-coronavirus-biden/2021/01/03/ea8902b0-3a39-11eb-98c4-25dc9f4987e8_story.html?_pml=1.
13. *USA Today* Staff, "Here's Everyone at the White House Rose Garden SCOTUS Event Now Called a Likely 'Superspreader.' Help Us ID Them All," *USA Today*,

January 28, 2021, https://www.usatoday.com/in-depth/news/investigations/2020/10/07/likely-rose-garden-covid-superspreader-white-house-drew-hundreds/3636925001/.

14. D. Leonhardt, "Red COVID," *New York Times*, September 27, 2021 (updated October 1, 2021), https://www.nytimes.com/2021/09/27/briefing/covid-red-states-vaccinations.html.

15. B. Franz and L. Y. Dhanani, "Beyond Political Affiliation: An Examination of the Relationships Between Social Factors and Perceptions of and Responses to COVID-19," *Journal of Behavioral Medicine* 44, no. 5 (2021): 641–52.

16. K. Collins et al., "Trump Picks Robert F. Kennedy Jr. to Be His Department of Health and Human Services Secretary," CNN, November 14, 2024, https://www.cnn.com/2024/11/14/politics/robert-f-kennedy-donald-trump-hhs/index.html; B. Lovelace and D. Weldon, "Trump's CDC Pick Could Bolster an RFK Jr. Anti-vaccine Agenda," NBC News, November 25, 2024, https://www.nbcnews.com/health/health-news/weldon-trump-cdc-rfk-jr-vaccine-children-rcna181701.

17. W. McDuffie et al., "RFK Jr.'s Lawyer and Top Ally Asked FDA to Revoke Approval of Polio Vaccine," ABC News, December 13, 2024, https://abcnews.go.com/Politics/rfk-jrs-lawyer-top-ally-asked-fda-revoke/story?id=116769906.

18. "CDC A(H5N1) Bird Flu Response Update November 18, 2024," Centers for Disease Control and Prevention, November 18, 2024, https://www.cdc.gov/bird-flu/spotlights/h5n1-response-11152024.html.

19. J. L. Graves and A. Goodman, *Racism, Not Race: Answers to Frequently Asked Questions* (Columbia University Press, 2022).

20. D. J. Downes et al., "Identification of LZTFL1 as a Candidate Effector Gene at a COVID-19 Risk Locus," *Nature Genetics* 53 (2021):1606–15, doi: 10.1038/s41588-021-00955-3.

21. D. Reich, *Who We Are and How We Got Here: Ancient DNA and the New Science of the Human Past* (Pantheon, 2018).

22. E. T. Norris et al., "Genetic Ancestry, Admixture and Health Determinants in Latin America," *BMC Genomics* 19 (2018):861, doi: 10.1186/s12864-018-5195-7.

23. G. H. L. Roberts et al., "Expanded COVID-19 Phenotype Definitions Reveal Distinct Patterns of Genetic Association and Protective Effects," *Nature Genetics* 54, no. 4 (2022): 374–81.

24. J. C. Knight, *Human Genetic Diversity: Functional Consequences for Health and Disease* (Oxford University Press, 2012).

25. S. Bunyavanich et al., "Racial/Ethnic Variation in Nasal Gene Expression of Transmembrane Serine Protease 2 (*TMPRSS2*)," *Journal of the American Medical Association* 324, no. 15 (2020): 1567–68.

26. J. Yuan et al., "Integrative Comparison of the Genomic and Transcriptomic Landscape Between Prostate Cancer Patients of Predominantly African or European Genetic Ancestry," *PLoS Genetics* 16, no. 2 (2020): e1008641.

27. N. Cifuentes-Munoz et al., "Viral Cell-to-Cell Spread: Conventional and Non-conventional Ways," *Advances in Virus Research* 108 (2020): 85–125.

28. O. Puhach et al., "SARS-CoV-2 Viral Load and Shedding Kinetics," *Nature Reviews Microbiology* 21 (2023): 147–61.

29. Y. Hou et al., "New Insights Into Genetic Susceptibility of COVID-19: An ACE2 and *TMPRSS2* Polymorphism Analysis," *BMC Medicine* 18, no. 1 (2020): 216.

30. C. de la Cova, "Race, Health, and Disease in 19th-Century-Born Males," *American Journal of Physical Anthropology* 144, no. 4 (2011): 526–37.

31. T. Rashburn and R. H. Steckel, "The Health of Slaves in the East" in *The Back Bone of History: Health and Nutrition in the Western Hemisphere*, ed. T. Rashburn and J. C. Rose (Cambridge University Press, 2002): 208–225.

32. J. Downs, *Sick from Freedom: African-American Illness and Suffering During the Civil War and Reconstruction* (Oxford University Press, 2012).
33. C. Lee, "Socioeconomic Differences in the Health of Black Union Soldiers During the American Civil War," *Social Science History* 33, no. 4 (2009): 427–57.
34. J. S. Sartin, "Infectious Diseases During the Civil War: The Triumph of the 'Third Army,'" *Clinical Infectious Disease* 16, no. 4 (1993): 580–84.
35. M. Humphries, *Intensely Human: The Health of the Black Soldier in the American Civil War* (John Hopkins University Press, 2008).
36. H. Aptheker, "Negro Causalities in the Civil War," *Journal of Negro History* 32, no. 1 (1947): 10–80.
37. Downs, *Sick from Freedom*.
38. J. L. Graves, *The Emperor's New Clothes: Biological Theories of Race at the Millennium* (Rutgers University Press, 2005).
39. C. Irmscher, *Louis Agassiz: Creator of American Science* (Houghton Mifflin Harcourt, 2013).
40. A. M. Brandt, "Racism and Research: The Case of the Tuskegee Syphilis Study," *Hastings Center Report* 8, no. 6 (1978): 21–29.
41. C. D. Willoughby, "Running Away from Drapetomania: Samuel A. Cartwright, Medicine, and Race in the Antebellum South," *Journal of Southern History* 84 (2018): 571–614.
42. D. P. Adams, *Foundations of Infectious Disease: A Public Health Perspective* (Jones & Bartlett Learning, 2021).
43. "Tuberculosis," World Health Organization, November 7, 2023, https://www.who.int /news-room/fact-sheets/detail/tuberculosis.
44. M. M. Torchia, "The Tuberculosis Movement and the Race Question, 1890–1950," *Bulletin of the History of Medicine* 49, no. 2 (1975): 152–68.
45. H. H. Hazen, "Syphilis in the American Negro," *Journal of the American Medical Association* 63, no. 6 (1914); W. T. English, "The Negro Problem from the Physician's Point of View," *Atlanta Journal Record of Medicine* 5 (1903): 461.
46. K. F. Maxcy and W. A. Brumfeld, "A Serological Survey for Syphilis in a Negro Population," *Southern Medical Journal* 27 (1934): 891–901.
47. J. H. Jones, *Bad Blood: The Tuskegee Syphilis Experiment* (Free Press, 1993).
48. Centers for Disease Control, "The US Public Health Service Untreated Syphilis Study at Tuskegee," September 4, 2024, https://www.cdc.gov/tuskegee/about/index.html.
49. Brandt, "Racism and Research."
50. R. M. White, "Unraveling the Tuskegee Study of Untreated Syphilis," *Archives of Internal Medicine* 160, no. 5 (2000): 585–98.
51. White, "Unraveling."
52. W. M. Cobb, "The Tuskegee Syphilis Study," *Journal of the National Medical Association* 65, no. 4 (1973): 345–48.
53. Committee on Science, Engineering, and Public Policy, *On Being a Scientist: A Guide to Responsible Conduct in Research*, 3rd ed. (National Academy of Sciences, National Academy of Engineering, Institute of Medicine, 2009), https://www.nationalacademies.org/our-work/on-being-a-scientist-a-guide-to-responsible-conduct-in-research -third-edition.
54. D. M. Hillis, "AIDS. Origins of HIV," *Science* 288, no. 5472 (2000): 1757–79.
55. N. R. Faria et al., "HIV Epidemiology. The Early Spread and Epidemic Ignition of HIV-1 in Human Populations," *Science* 346, no. 6205 (2014): 56–61.
56. M. Worobey et al., "Direct Evidence of Extensive Diversity of HIV-1 in Kinshasa by 1960," *Nature* 455, no. 7213 (2008): 661–64.

57. G. J. Bell et al., "Race, Place, and HIV: The Legacies of Apartheid and Racist Policy in South Africa," *Social Science & Medicine* 296 (2022): 114755.

58. W. D. Johnson Jr. and J. W. Pape, "AIDS in Haiti," *Immunology Series* 44 (1989): 65–78.

59. M. T. Gilbert et al., "The Emergence of HIV/AIDS in the Americas and Beyond," *Proceedings of the National Academy of Sciences of the United States of America* 104, no. 47 (2007): 18566–70.

60. P. Farmer, *AIDS and Accusation* (University of California Press, 2006); J. Cohen, "HIV/AIDS: Latin America & Caribbean. Haiti: Making Headway Under Hellacious Circumstances," *Science* 313, no. 5786 (2006): 470–73.

61. K. A. Bosh et al., "Estimated Annual Number of HIV Infections—United States, 1981–2019," *Morbidity and Mortality Weekly Report* 70, no. 22 (2021): 801–806.

62. Bosh et al., "Estimated Annual Number of HIV Infections."

63. D. C. Lemly et al., "Race and Sex Differences in Antiretroviral Therapy Use and Mortality Among HIV-Infected Persons in Care," *Journal of Infectious Diseases* 199, no. 7 (2009): 991–98.

64. M. Aziz and K. Y. Smith, "Challenges and Successes in Linking HIV-Infected Women to Care in the United States," *Clinical Infectious Diseases* 52, no. S2 (2011): S231–37.

65. W. E. Du Bois, "The Health and Physique of the Negro American. 1906," *American Journal of Public Health* 93, no. 2 (2003): 272–76.

66. W. M. Cobb, *Medical Care and the Plight of the Negro* (National Association for the Advancement of Colored People, 1947).

67. B. D. Smedley et al., eds., *Unequal Treatment: Confronting Racial and Ethnic Disparities in Health Care* (National Institutes of Medicine, 2003).

68. A. Li et al., "Race in the Reading: A Study of Problematic Uses of Race and Ethnicity in a Prominent Pediatrics Textbook," *Academic Medicine* 97, no. 10 (2022): 1521–27.

6. BAD BLOOD: THE RACIALIZATION OF SICKLE CELL ANEMIA

1. T. L. Savitt and M. F. Goldberg, "Herrick's 1910 Case Report of Sickle Cell Anemia. The Rest of the Story," *Journal of the American Medical Association* 261, no. 2 (1989): 266–71; G. R. Serjeant, "One Hundred Years of Sickle Cell Disease," *British Journal of Haematology* 151, no. 5 (2010): 425–29.

2. T. L. Savitt, "The Second Reported Case of Sickle Cell Anemia. Charlottesville, Virginia, 1911," *Virginia Medical Quarterly* 124, no. 2 (1997): 84–92.

3. J. E. Cook and J. Meyer, "Severe Anemia with Remarkable Elongated and Sickle-Shaped Red Blood Cells and Chronic Leg Ulcers," *Archives of Internal Medicine* 16 (1915): 644–51.

4. V. R. Mason, "Landmark Article Oct. 14, 1922: Sickle Cell Anemia. By V. R. Mason," *Journal of the American Medical Association* 254, no. 14 (1985): 1955–57.

5. K. Wailoo, "Genetic Marker of Segregation: Sickle Cell Anemia, Thalassemia, and Racial Ideology in American Medical Writing 1920–1950," *History and Philosophy of the Life Sciences* 18, no. 3 (1996): 305–20.

6. J. L. Graves, "Genetics and American Science," in *The Routledge History of American Science*, ed. T. Kneeland (Routledge, 2023).

7. J. L. Graves, *The Emperor's New Clothes: Biological Theories of Race at the Millennium* (Rutgers University Press, 2005).

8. F. Clarke, "Sickle Cell Anemia in the White Race with Report of Two Cases," *Nebraska Medical Journal* 18 (1923): 376–79.

9. "Sickle Cell Anemia, a Race Specific Disease," *Journal of the American Medical Association* 133 (1947): 33–34.

10. A. W. F. Edwards, "G. H. Hardy (1908) and Hardy–Weinberg Equilibrium," *Genetics* 179, no. 3 (2008): 1143–50.

11. W. B. Provine, *The Origins of Theoretical Population Genetics* (University of Chicago Press, 1991).

12. R. A. Fisher, *The Genetical Theory of Natural Selection* (Clarendon, 1931).

13. Wailoo, "Genetic Marker of Segregation."

14. G. Serjeant, *Sickle Cell Disease* (Oxford University Press, 1985).

15. J. V. Neel, "The Inheritance of Sickle Cell Anemia," *Science* 110, no. 2846 (1949): 64–66; E. A. Beet, "The Genetics of the Sickle-Cell Trait in a Bantu Tribe," *Annals of Eugenics* 14, no. 4 (1949): 279–84.

16. Sergeant, *Sickle Cell Disease.*

17. L. Pauling et al., "Sickle Cell Anemia a Molecular Disease," *Science* 110, no. 2865 (1949): 543–48.

18. D. Paul, "From Eugenics to Medical Genetics," *Journal of Policy History* 9, no. 1 (1997): 96–116.

19. Sergeant, *Sickle Cell Disease.*

20. H. Lehman and A. B. Raper, "Maintenance of High Sickling Rate in an African Community," *British Medical Journal* 2, no. 4988 (1956): 333–36.

21. T. Dobzhansky, *Genetics and the Origin of Species* (Columbia University Press, 1951).

22. S. Fan et al., "Going Global by Adapting Local: A Review of Recent Human Adaptation," *Science* 354, no. 6308 (2016): 54–59; C. López et al., "Mechanisms of Genetically Based Resistance to Malaria," *Gene* 467, nos. 1–2 (2010): 1–12.

23. S. H. Orkin and H. H. Kazazian Jr., "Mutation and Polymorphism of the Human Beta-Globin Gene and Its Surrounding DNA," *Annual Review of Genetics* 18 (1984): 131–71.

24. L. C. Foo et al., "Ovalocytosis Protects Against Severe Malaria Parasitemia in the Malayan Aborigines," *American Journal of Tropical Medicine and Hygiene* 47, no. 3 (1992): 271–75.

25. C. Garnett and B. J. Bain, "South-East Asian Ovalocytosis," *American Journal of Hematology* 88, no. 4 (2013): 328.

26. M. D. Cappellini and G. Fiorelli, "Glucose-6-Phosphate Dehydrogenase Deficiency," *Lancet* 371 (2008): 64–74.

27. L. Luzzatto et al., "Glucose-6-Phosphate Dehydrogenase Deficiency," *Blood* 136, no. 11 (2020): 1225–40.

28. C. M. Mann, *1493: Uncovering the New World That Columbus Created* (Vintage, 2011).

29. J. M. Gonzalez Sepulveda et al., "Preferences for Potential Benefits and Risks for Gene Therapy in the Treatment of Sickle Cell Disease," *Blood Advances* 7, no. 23 (2023): 7371–81.

30. Sergeant, *Sickle Cell Disease.*

31. L. A. Smith et al., "Sickle Cell Disease: A Question of Equity and Quality," *Pediatrics* 117, no. 5 (2006): 1763–70.

32. K. Wailoo, "Sickle Cell Disease – A History of Progress and Peril," *New England Journal of Medicine* 376, no. 9 (2017): 805–807; D. Anderson et al., "The Bias of Medicine in Sickle Cell Disease," *Journal of General Internal Medicine* 38, no. 14 (2023): 3247–51.

33. Anderson et al., "The Bias of Medicine."

34. A. M. Brandow et al., "American Society of Hematology 2020 Guidelines for Sickle Cell Disease: Management of Acute and Chronic Pain," *Blood Advances* 4, no. 12 (2020): 2656–701.

35. C. L. Dean et al., "Multiple Hemolytic Transfusion Reactions Misinterpreted as Severe Vaso-occlusive Crisis in a Patient with Sickle Cell Disease," *Transfusion* 59, no. 2 (2019): 448–53.

36. K. M. Hoffman et al., "Racial Bias in Pain Assessment and Treatment Recommendations, and False Beliefs About Biological Differences Between Blacks and Whites," *Proceedings of the National Academy of Sciences of the United States of America* 113, no. 16 (2016): 4296–301.

37. N. S. Ruta and S. K. Ballas, "The Opioid Drug Epidemic and Sickle Cell Disease: Guilt by Association," *Pain Medicine* 17, no. 10 (2016): 1793–98.

38. V. Scotet et al., "The Changing Epidemiology of Cystic Fibrosis: Incidence, Survival and Impact of the *CFTR* Gene Discovery," *Genes* 11, no. 6 (2020): 589.

39. F. Farooq et al., "Comparison of US Federal and Foundation Funding of Research for Sickle Cell Disease and Cystic Fibrosis and Factors Associated with Research Productivity," *JAMA Network Open* 3, no. 3 (2020): e201737.

40. "Hemophilia Treatment Center (HTC) Directory," Centers for Disease Control and Prevention, accessed June 3, 2024, https://dbdgateway.cdc.gov/HTCDirSearch.aspx.

41. A. Grady et al., "Profile of Medicaid Enrollees with Sickle Cell Disease: A High Need, High Cost Population," *PLoS One* 16, no. 10 (2021): e0257796.

42. L. Ma et al., "CRISPR/Cas9-Based Gene-Editing Technology for Sickle Cell Disease," *Gene* 874 (2023): 147480.

43. J. W. R. Sins et al., "Pharmacotherapeutical Strategies in the Prevention of Acute, Vaso-occlusive Pain in Sickle Cell Disease: A Systematic Review," *Blood Advances* 1, no. 19 (2017): 1598–1616.

44. I. Osunkwo et al., "Current and Novel Therapies for the Prevention of Vaso-occlusive Crisis in Sickle Cell Disease," *Therapeutic Advances in Hematology* 11 (2020): 2040620720955000.

45. J. A. Doudna and E. Charpentier, "Genome Editing. The New Frontier of Genome Engineering with CRISPR-Cas9," *Science* 346, no. 6213 (2014): 1258096.

46. E. S. Lander et al., "Adopt a Moratorium on Heritable Genome Editing," *Nature* 567, no. 7747 (2019): 165–68.

47. E. Boodman, "Coercive Care, A STAT Investigation: How Doctors Are Pressuring Sickle Cell Patients Into Unwanted Sterilizations," *STAT*, May 21, 2024, https://www.statnews.com/2024/05/21/sickle-cell-patients-steered-toward-sterilization-for-decades/.

48. Ma et al., "CRISPR/Cas9-Based Gene-Editing Technology."

49. H. Frangoul et al., "CRISPR-Cas9 Gene Editing for Sickle Cell Disease and β-Thalassemia," *New England Journal of Medicine* 384, no. 3 (2021): 252–60; A. Sharma et al., "CRISPR-Cas9 Editing of the *HBG1* and *HBG2* Promoters to Treat Sickle Cell Disease," *New England Journal of Medicine* 389, no. 9 (2023): 820–32.

50. B. R. Sanders et al., "Reporting Off-Target Effects of Recombinant Engineering Using the pORTMAGE System," *Journal of Microbiological Methods* 204 (2023): 106627.

51. Frangoul et al., "CRISPR-Cas9 Gene Editing"; Ma et al., "CRISPR/Cas9-Based Gene-Editing Technology"; Sharma et al., "CRISPR-Cas9 Editing."

52. K. Lin, "Will the High Price of Gene Therapy for Sickle Cell Disease Put This Cure Out of Reach?," American Family Physician Community Blog, December 12, 2023, https://www.aafp.org/pubs/afp/afp-community-blog/entry/will-the-high-price-of-gene -therapy-for-sickle-cell-disease-put-this-cure-out-of-reach.html.

53. "Biden–Harris Administration Announces Action to Increase Access to Sickle Cell Disease Treatments," Centers for Medicare & Medicaid Services, January 30, 2024, https://www.cms.gov/newsroom/press-releases/biden-harris-administration-announces -action-increase-access-sickle-cell-disease-treatments.

54. US HHS, HHS Announces Transformation to Make America Healthy Again, March 27, 2025, accessed April 15, 202,5 https://www.hhs.gov/press-room/hhs-restructuring-doge .html.

7. CANCER IS UNFAIR

1. W. R. Clark, A Means to an End: The Biological Basis of Aging and Death (Oxford University Press, 1999).

2. S. Stearns and R. Medzhitov, Evolutionary Medicine (Sinauer, 2016); R. Janivara and J. Lachance, "The Genetic Hitchhiker's Guide to Tumor Evolution," in Cancer Through the Lens of Evolution and Ecology, ed. J. Somarelli and N. A. Johnson (CRC, 2024).

3. S. Shostak and M. Bentley, hosts and producers, Big Picture Science, podcast, "Going Multicellular," October 9, 2023, https://bigpicturescience.org/episodes/going-multicellular.

4. M. D. Herron et al., eds. The Evolution of Multicellularity (CRC, 2022).

5. A. Burnetti and W. C. Ratcliff, "Experimental Evolution Is not Just for Model Organisms," PLoS Biology 20, no. 3 (2022): e3001587.

6. C. Yao and J. M. Billette, "Short-Term Cancer Prevalence in Canada, 2018," Health Reports 33, no. 3 (2022): 15–21.

7. K. Hill, "The Demography of Menopause," Maturitas 23, no. 2 (1996): 113–27.

8. L. D. Mueller et al., "The Death Spiral: Predicting Death in Drosophila Cohorts," Biogerontology 17, nos. 5–6 (2016): 805–16.

9. A. Scally and R. Durbin, "Revising the Human Mutation Rate: Implications for Understanding Human Evolution," Nature Reviews Genetics 13, no. 10 (2012): 745–53.

10. R. Halliburton, Introduction to Population Genetics (Prentice Hall, 2004).

11. K. R. Arnold and M. R. Rose, Conceptual Breakthroughs in the Evolutionary Biology of Aging (Academic, 2023).

12. American Cancer Society, Cancer Facts & Figures 2024 (American Cancer Society, 2024), https://www.cancer.org/content/dam/cancer-org/research/cancer-facts-and-statistics /annual-cancer-facts-and-figures/2024/2024-cancer-facts-and-figures-acs.pdf.

13. D. Hoyos et al., "The Genotypes and Phenotypes of Missense Mutations in the Proline Domain of the p53 Protein," Cell Death and Differentiation 29, no. 5 (2022): 938–45.

14. J. Rhee et al., "Serum Concentrations of Per- and Polyfluoroalkyl Substances and Risk of Renal Cell Carcinoma in the Multiethnic Cohort Study," Environment International 180 (2023): 108197.

15. R. D. Bullard et al., Toxic Wastes and Race at Twenty: 1987–2007 (United Church of Christ, 2007), https://www.ucc.org/what-we-do/justice-local-church-ministries/efam /environmental-justice/environmental-ministries_toxic-waste-20/.

16. B. Woo et al., "Residential Segregation and Racial/Ethnic Disparities in Ambient Air Pollution," Race and Social Problems 11, no. 1 (2019): 60–67.

17. H. Landrine et al., "Residential Segregation and Racial Cancer Disparities: A Systematic Review," *Journal of Racial and Ethnic Health Disparities* 4, no. 6 (2017): 1195–1205.

18. K. Voskarides and N. Giannopoulou, "The Role of *TP53* in Adaptation and Evolution," *Cells* 12, no. 3 (2023): 512.

19. B. Möller et al., "Expression of the Angiogenic Growth Factors VEGF, FGF-2, EGF and Their Receptors in Normal Human Endometrium During the Menstrual Cycle," *Molecular Human Reproduction* 7, no. 1 (2001): 65–72.

20. Voskarides and Giannopoulou, "The Role of *TP53*."

21. M. K. Schmidt et al., "Combined Effects of Single Nucleotide Polymorphisms TP53 R72P and MDM2 SNP309, and p53 Expression on Survival of Breast Cancer Patients," *Breast Cancer Research* 11, no. 6 (2009): R89.

22. M. Roginski et al., "Paradoxes of Breast Cancer Incidence and Mortality in Two Corners of Europe," *BMC Cancer* 22, no. 1 (2022): 1123; A. Barchuk et al., "Breast and Cervical Cancer Incidence and Mortality Trends in Russia 1980–2013," *Cancer Epidemiology* 55 (2018): 73–80.

23. L. Moore et al., "The Mutational Landscape of Human Somatic and Germline Cells," *Nature* 597, no. 7876 (2021): 381–86.

24. E. Weiderpass et al., "Breast Cancer and Occupational Exposures in Women in Finland," *American Journal of Industrial Medicine* 36, no. 1 (1999): 48–53.

25. Global Burden of Disease Cancer Collaboration et al., "The Global Burden of Cancer 2013," *JAMA Oncology* 1, no. 4 (2015): 505–27.

26. J. L. Graves and A. Goodman, *Racism, Not Race: Answers to Frequently Asked Questions* (Columbia University Press, 2022).

27. D. J. Taylor et al., "Sources of Gene Expression Variation in a Globally Diverse Human Cohort," *Nature* 632 (2024): 122–30.

28. A. N. Giaquinto et al., "Breast Cancer Statistics, 2022," *CA: A Cancer Journal for Clinicians* 72, no. 6 (2022): 524–41.

29. F. Islami et al., "Proportion and Number of Cancer Cases and Deaths Attributable to Potentially Modifiable Risk Factors in the United States," *CA: A Cancer Journal for Clinicians* 68, no. 1 (2018): 31–54.

30. Giaguinto et al., "Breast Cancer Statistics, 2022."

31. J. L. Graves, "The Costs of Reproduction and Dietary Restriction in Mammals," *Growth, Development, and Aging* 57, no. 4 (1993): 233–49.

32. H. Sung et al., "Breast Cancer Subtypes Among Eastern-African-Born Black Women and Other Black Women in the United States," *Cancer* 125, no. 19 (2019): 3401–11.

33. S. J. Micheletti et al., "Genetic Consequences of the Transatlantic Slave Trade in the Americas," *American Journal of Human Genetics* 107, no. 2 (2020): 265–77.

34. All of Us Research Program Genomics Investigators, "Genomic Data in the All of Us Research Program," *Nature* 627, no. 8003 (2024): 340–46.

35. E. Linnenbringer et al., "Associations Between Breast Cancer Subtype and Neighborhood Socioeconomic and Racial Composition Among Black and White Women," *Breast Cancer Research and Treatment* 180, no. 2 (2020): 437–47.

36. Giaguinto et al., "Breast Cancer Statistics, 2022."

37. I. Jatoi et al., "The Emergence of the Racial Disparity in U.S. Breast-Cancer Mortality," *New England Journal of Medicine* 386, no. 25 (2022): 2349–52.

38. L. J. Collin et al., "Neighborhood-Level Redlining and Lending Bias Are Associated with Breast Cancer Mortality in a Large and Diverse Metropolitan Area," *Cancer Epidemiology, Biomarkers & Prevention* 30, no. 1 (2021): 53–60.

8. RACE AND EPIGENOMICS:
NOBODY KNOWS THE TROUBLE WE'VE SEEN

1. N. Snyder-Mackler et al., "Social Determinants of Health and Survival in Humans and Other Animals," *Science* 368, no. 6493 (2020): eaax9553.

2. V. Kumar, et al., eds., *Robbins Basic Pathology*, 10th ed. (Elsevier, 2017).

3. See, for example, J. L. Graves and A. Goodman, *Racism, Not Race: Answers to Frequently Asked Questions* (Columbia University Press, 2022), chap. 4, 5.

4. M. D. Thomas et al., "Too Much of a Good Thing: Adaptation to Iron (II) Intoxication in *Escherichia coli*," *Evolution, Medicine, and Public Health* 9, no. 1 (2021): 53–57.

5. J. Casadesús and D. A. Low, "Programmed Heterogeneity: Epigenetic Mechanisms in Bacteria," *Journal of Biological Chemistry* 288, no. 20 (2013): 13929–35; D. Ghosh et al., "Antibiotic Resistance and Epigenetics: More to It Than Meets the Eye," *Antimicrobial Agents and Chemotherapy* 64, no. 2 (2020): e02225-19.

6. T. T. Barter et al., "*Drosophila* Transcriptomics with and Without Ageing," *Biogerontology* 20, no. 5 (2019): 699–710.

7. S.-E. Cardin and G. M. Borchert, "Viral MicroRNAs, Host MicroRNAs Regulating Viruses, and Bacterial MicroRNA-Like RNAs," *Methods in Molecular Biology* 1617 (2017): 39–56.

8. A. J. Bannister and T. Kouzarides, "Regulation of Chromatin by Histone Modifications," *Cell Research* 21, no. 3 (2011): 381–95.

9. C. L. Martin et al., "Understanding Health Inequalities Through the Lens of Social Epigenetics," *Annual Review of Public Health* 43 (2022): 235–54.

10. A. T. Geronimus, *Weathering: The Extraordinary Stress of Ordinary Life in an Unjust Society* (Little, Brown, Spark, 2023); N. Krieger, *Epidemiology and the People's Health: Theory and Context*, 2nd ed. (Oxford University Press, 2024).

11. E. Arias et al., "Provisional Life Expectancy Estimates for January Through June, 2020," *Vital Statistics Rapid Release*, Report No. 10 (2021); J. A. Martin et al., "Births: Final Data for 2019," *National Vital Statistics Report* 70, no. 2 (2019).

12. Martin et al., "Understanding Health Inequalities."

13. "Epigenetics and Methylation Analysis," Oxford Nanopore Technologies, accessed June 10, 2024, https://nanoporetech.com/applications/investigations/epigenetics-and -methylation-analysis.

14. I. S. Kiselev et al., "DNA Methylation as an Epigenetic Mechanism in the Development of Multiple Sclerosis," *Acta Naturae* 13, no. 2 (2021): 45–57.

15. M. E. Levine, "Assessment of Epigenetic Clocks as Biomarkers of Aging in Basic and Population Research," *Journals of Gerontology Series A: Biological Sciences and Medical Sciences* 75, no. 3 (2020): 463–65.

16. S. Frenk and J. Houseley, "Gene Expression Hallmarks of Cellular Ageing," *Biogerontology* 19, no. 6 (2018): 547–66; R. Yamamoto et al., "Tissue-Specific Impacts of Aging and Genetics on Gene Expression Patterns in Humans," *Nature Communications* 13, no. 1 (2022): 5803.

17. E. Arias and J. Xu, "United States Life Tables, 2015," *National Vital Statistics Reports* 67, no. 7 (2018), https://www.cdc.gov/nchs/data/nvsr/nvsr67/nvsr67_07-508.pdf.

18. K. M. Hoffman et al., "Racial Bias in Pain Assessment and Treatment Recommendations, and False Beliefs About Biological Differences Between Blacks and Whites," *Proceedings of the National Academy of Sciences of the United States of America* 113, no. 16 (2016): 4296–301.

19. Graves and Goodman, *Racism, Not Race.*

20. S. M. Tajuddin et al., "Novel Age-Associated DNA Methylation Changes and Epigenetic Age Acceleration in Middle-Aged African Americans and Whites," *Clinical Epigenetics* 11, no. 1 (2019): 119; N. Noren Hooten et al., "The Accelerated Aging Phenotype: The Role of Race and Social Determinants of Health on Aging," *Ageing Research Reviews* 73 (2022): 101536.

21. K. N. Chitrala et al., "Race-Specific Alterations in DNA Methylation Among Middle-Aged African Americans and Whites with Metabolic Syndrome," *Epigenetics* 15, no. 5 (2020): 462–82.

22. S. C. Hunt et al., "Leukocyte Telomeres Are Longer in African Americans than in Whites: The National Heart, Lung, and Blood Institute Family Heart Study and the Bogalusa Heart Study," *Aging Cell* 7, no. 4 (2008): 451–58; M. Rewak et al., "Race-Related Health Disparities and Biological Aging: Does Rate of Telomere Shortening Differ Across Blacks and Whites?," *Biological Psychology* 99 (2014): 92–99.

23. See the discussion of maternal effects and selection in D. S. Falconer and T. Mackay, introduction to *Quantitative Genetics*, 4th ed. (Longman, 1996: 199, 212). See also J. K. Abbott, "Epigenetics and Sex-Specific Fitness: An Experimental Test Using Male-Limited Evolution in *Drosophila melanogaster*," *PLoS One* 8, no. 7 (2013): e70493.

24. Z. D. Smith et al., "A Unique Regulatory Phase of DNA Methylation in the Early Mammalian Embryo," *Nature* 484, no. 7394 (2012): 339–44; R. Xu et al., "Insights Into Epigenetic Patterns in Mammalian Early Embryos," *Protein & Cell* 12, no. 1 (2021): 7–28.

25. J. R. McCarrey, "Distinctions Between Transgenerational and Non-transgenerational Epimutations," *Molecular and Cellular Endocrinology* 398, nos. 1–2 (2014): 13–23; M. H. Fitz-James and G. Cavalli, "Molecular Mechanisms of Transgenerational Epigenetic Inheritance," *Nature Reviews Genetics* 23, no. 6 (2022): 325–41.

26. G. Turecki and M. J. Meaney, "Effects of the Social Environment and Stress on Glucocorticoid Receptor Gene Methylation: A Systematic Review," *Biological Psychiatry* 79, no. 2 (2016): 87–96.

27. S. R. Moore et al., "Infant DNA Methylation: An Early Indicator of Intergenerational Trauma?," *Early Human Development* 164 (2022): 105519.

28. A. E. Shields et al., "Childhood Abuse, Promoter Methylation of Leukocyte NR3C1 and the Potential Modifying Effect of Emotional Support," *Epigenomics* 8, no. 11 (2016): 1507–17.

29. S. M. Kogan et al., "Oxytocin Receptor Gene Methylation and Substance Use Problems Among Young African American Men," *Drug and Alcohol Dependence* 192 (2018): 309–15.

30. C. L. Martin et al., "Understanding Health Inequalities"; N. Noren Hooten, "The Accelerated Aging Phenotype: The Role of Race and Social Determinants of Health on Aging," *Ageing Research Reviews* 73 (2022): 101536.

31. R. J. David and J. W. Collins Jr., "Differing Birth Weight Among Infants of U.S.-Born Blacks, African-Born Blacks, and U.S.-Born Whites," *New England Journal of Medicine* 337, no. 17 (1997): 1209–14.

32. H. M. Salihu et al., "Racial Differences in DNA-Methylation of CpG Sites Within Preterm-Promoting Genes and Gene Variants," *Maternal and Child Health Journal* 20, no. 8 (2016): 1680–87.

33. C. L. Martin et al., "Understanding Health Inequalities."

34. K. Kirkinis et al., "Racism, Racial Discrimination, and Trauma: A Systematic Review of the Social Science Literature," *Ethnicity & Health* 26, no. 3 (2021): 392–412.

35. G. M. Babulal et al., "Perspectives on Ethnic and Racial Disparities in Alzheimer's Disease and Related Dementias: Update and Areas of Immediate Need," *Alzheimer's & Dementia* 15, no. 2 (2019): 292–312.

36. A. Elbasheir et al., "Racial Discrimination, Neural Connectivity, and Epigenetic Aging Among Black Women," *JAMA Network Open* 7, no. 6 (2024): e2416588.

37. S. S. Shiek et al., "Health Repercussions of Environmental Exposure to Lead: Methylation Perspective," *Toxicology* 461 (2021): 152927.

38. Centers for Disease Control and Prevention, Blood Lead Levels—United States, 1999–2002," *Morbidity and Mortality Weekly Report* 54, no. 20 (2005): 513–16.

39. M. L. Miranda et al., "Segregation and Childhood Blood Lead Levels in North Carolina," *Pediatrics* 152, no. 3 (2023): e2022058661.

40. N. Vilahur et al., "The Epigenetic Effects of Prenatal Cadmium Exposure," *Current Environmental Health Reports* 2, no. 2 (2015): 195–203; F. Khan et al., "The Relationship Between Mercury Exposure and Epigenetic Alterations Regarding Human Health, Risk Assessment and Diagnostic Strategies," *Journal of Trace Elements in Medicine and Biology* 52 (2019): 37–47; S. Kim et al., "Epigenetic Changes by Per- and Polyfluoroalkyl Substances (PFAS)," *Environmental Pollution* 279 (2021): 116929.

41. R. D. Bullard et al., *Toxic Wastes and Race at Twenty, 1987–2007* (United Church of Christ, 2007), https://www.ucc.org/what-we-do/justice-local-church-ministries/efam/environmental-justice/environmental-ministries_toxic-waste-20/.

42. As discussed in J. L. Graves, "Looking at the World Through Race-Colored Glasses: The Influence of Ascertainment Bias on Biomedical Research and Practice," in *Mapping "Race": A Critical Reader on Health Disparities Research*, ed. L. Gomez and N. Lopez (Rutgers University Press, 2013: 39–52).

43. S. Lindeberg, *Food and Western Disease: Health and Nutrition from an Evolutionary Perspective* (Wiley-Blackwell, 2009).

44. J. S. Bernal et al., "Did Maize Domestication and Early Spread Mediate the Population Genetics of Corn Leafhopper?," *Insect Science* 26, no. 3 (2019): 569–86; C. Burgarella et al., "A Western Sahara Centre of Domestication Inferred from Pearl Millet Genomes," *Nature Ecology & Evolution* 2, no. 9 (2018): 1377–80.

45. M. Dehghan et al., "Associations of Fats and Carbohydrate Intake with Cardiovascular Disease and Mortality in 18 Countries from Five Continents (PURE): A Prospective Cohort Study," *Lancet* 390, no. 10107 (2017): 2050–62.

46. R. M. Nesse, *Good Reasons for Bad Feelings: Insights from the Frontiers of Evolutionary Psychiatry* (Dutton, 2019); M. A. Rossi and G. D. Stuber, "Overlapping Brain Circuits for Homeostatic and Hedonic Feeding," *Cell Metabolism* 27, no. 1 (2018): 42–56.

47. T. W. Davies et al., "Incidence of Myocardial Infarction Correlated with Venous and Pulmonary Thrombosis and Embolism. A Geographic Study Based on Autopsies in Uganda, East Africa and St. Louis, USA," *American Journal of Cardiology* 5 (1960): 41–47.

48. F. P. Cappuccio, "Epidemiologic Transition, Migration, and CVD," *International Journal of Epidemiology* 33 (2004): 387–88.

49. M. Wang et al., "Validation of a Genome-Wide Polygenic Score for Coronary Artery Disease in South Asians," *Journal of the American College of Cardiology* 76, no. 6 (2020): 703–14.

50. S. M. Damrauer et al., "Association of the V122I Hereditary Transthyretin Amyloidosis Genetic Variant with Heart Failure Among Individuals of African or Hispanic/Latino Ancestry," *Journal of the American Medical Association* 322, no. 22 (2019): 2191–202.

51. V. Kumar, A. Abbas, J. Aster, A. Deyrup, A. Das, *Robbins & Kumar: Basic Pathology*, 11th ed. (Elsevier, 2023).

52. Y. V. Sun et al., "Cardiovascular Disease Risk and Pathophysiology in South Asians: Can Longitudinal Multi-omics Shed Light?," *Wellcome Open Research* 5 (2021): 255.

53. J. Erdmann et al., "A Decade of Genome-Wide Association Studies for Coronary Artery Disease: The Challenges Ahead," *Cardiovascular Research* 114, no. 9 (2018): 1241–57.

54. J. L. M. Björkegren et al., "Genome-wide significant loci: how important are they? Systems genetics to understand heritability of coronary artery disease and other common complex disorders," *Journal of the American College of Cardiology* 65, no. 8 (2015): 830–45.

55. G. Agha et al., "Blood Leukocyte DNA Methylation Predicts Risk of Future Myocardial Infarction and Coronary Heart Disease," *Circulation* 140, no. 8 (2019): 645–57.

56. G. L. Wojcik et al., "Genetic Analyses of Diverse Populations Improves Discovery for Complex Traits," *Nature* 570, no. 7762 (2019): 514–18.

57. Y. Xia et al., "DNA Methylation Signatures of Incident Coronary Heart Disease: Findings from Epigenome-Wide Association Studies," *Clinical Epigenetics* 13, no. 1 (2021): 186.

58. A. S. Kong et al., "miRNA in Ischemic Heart Disease and Its Potential as Biomarkers: A Comprehensive Review," *International Journal of Molecular Science* 23, no. 16 (2022): 9001.

9. HOW ALGORITHMS CAN HURT

1. J. Huxley, "Clines: An Auxiliary Taxonomic Principle," *Nature* 142 (1938): 219–20.

2. J. Huxley and A. C. Haddon, *We Europeans: A Survey of Racial Problems* (Harper, 1936).

3. F. Livingston, "On the Non-existence of Human Races," *Current Anthropology* 3, no. 3 (1962): 279.

4. C. L. Brace, "A Non-racial Approach Towards the Understanding of Human Diversity," in *The Concept of Race*, ed. M. F. A. Montagu (Free Press, 1964: 313–20).

5. C. L. Brace, *"Race" Is a Four-Letter Word: The Genesis of the Concept* (Oxford University Press, 2005).

6. A. R. Templeton, "Biological Races in Humans," *Studies in History and Philosophy of Biological and Biomedical Sciences* 44, no. 3 (2013): 262–71.

7. L. L. Cavalli-Sforza and A. W. F. Edwards, "Analysis of Human Evolution," *Proceedings of the 11th International Congress of Genetics* 2 (1964): 923–33.

8. J. Raff, *Origin: A Genetic History of the Americas* (Hachette, 2023).

9. J. R. Golbus et al., "Wearable Device Signals and Home Blood Pressure Data Across Age, Sex, Race, Ethnicity, and Clinical Phenotypes in the Michigan Predictive Activity & Clinical Trajectories in Health (MIPACT) Study: A Prospective, Community-Based Observational Study," *Lancet Digital Health* 3, no. 11 (2021): e707–15.

10. Golbus et al., "Wearable Device Signals," e712.

11. M. Anderson, A Rising Share of the U.S. Black Population Is Foreign Born: 9 Percent Are Immigrants; and While Most Are from the Caribbean, Africans Drive Recent Growth (Pew Research Center, 2015), https://www.pewresearch.org/social -trends/2015/04/09/a-rising-share-of-the-u-s-black-population-is-foreign-born/.

12. R. Benjamin, *Race After Technology: Abolitionist Tools for the New Jim Code* (Polity, 2019).

13. L. Braun, "Race Correction and Spirometry: Why History Matters," *Chest* 159, no. 4 (2021): 1670–75.

14. J. L. Graves, *The Emperor's New Clothes: Biological Theories of Race at the Millennium* (Rutgers University Press, 2005).

15. A. Getu, "Ethiopian Native Highlander's Adaptation to Chronic High-Altitude Hypoxia," *BioMed Research International* 2022 (2022): 5749382.

16. N. R. Bhakta et al., "Addressing Race in Pulmonary Function Testing by Aligning Intent and Evidence with Practice and Perception," *Chest* 161, no. 1 (2022): 288–97.

17. B. J. Delgado and T. Bajaj, *Physiology, Lung Capacity* (StatPearls, 2023), https://www.ncbi.nlm.nih.gov/books/NBK541029/.

18. K. Wailoo, *Pushing Cool: Big Tobacco, Racial Marketing, and the Untold Story of the Menthol Cigarette* (University of Chicago Press, 2021); S. N. Bonner and E. Wakeam, "The End of Race Correction in Spirometry for Pulmonary Function Testing and Surgical Implications," *Annals of Surgery* 276, no. 1 (2022): e3–5; N. W. White, "'Ethic Discounting' and Spirometry," *Respiratory Medicine* 89, no. 4 (1995): 312–13; J. L. Graves and A. Goodman, *Racism, Not Race: Answers to Frequently Asked Questions* (Columbia University Press, 2022).

19. A. D. Baugh et al., "Reconsidering the Utility of Race-Specific Lung Function Prediction Equations," *American Journal of Respiratory and Critical Care Medicine* 205, no. 7 (2022): 819–29; erratum in *American Journal of Respiratory and Critical Care Medicine* 206, no. 2 (2022): 230.

20. House Committee on Ways and Means, *Fact Versus Fiction: Clinical Decision Support Tools and the (Mis)use of Race: Majority Staff Report* (House Committee on Ways and Means, 2021), https://democrats-waysandmeans.house.gov/sites/evo-subsites/democrats-waysandmeans.house.gov/files/documents/Fact%20Versus%20Fiction%20Clinical%20Decision%20Support%20Tools%20and%20the%20(Mis)Use%20of%20Race%20(2).pdf.

21. C. F. Vogelmeier et al., "Global Strategy for the Diagnosis, Management, and Prevention of Chronic Obstructive Lung Disease 2017 Report. GOLD Executive Summary." *American Journal of Respiratory Critical Care Medicine* 195, no. 5 (2017): 557–82.

22. W. D. Leslie and ASBMR Task Force on Clinical Algorithms for Fracture Risk, "Effect of Race/Ethnicity on United States FRAX Calculations and Treatment Qualification: A Registry-Based Study," *Journal of Bone and Mineral Research* 38, no. 12 (2023): 1742–48.

23. B. Dawson-Hughes et al., "Implications of Absolute Fracture Risk Assessment for Osteoporosis Practice Guidelines in the USA," *Osteoporosis International* 19, no. 4 (2008): 449–58.

24. M. Trotter et al., "Densities of Bones of White and Negro Skeletons," *Journal of Bone and Joint Surgery* 42-A (1960): 50–58.

25. S. J. Micheletti et al., "Genetic Consequences of the Transatlantic Slave Trade in the Americas," *American Journal of Human Genetics* 107, no. 2 (2020): 265–77.

26. K. Bryc et al., "The Genetic Ancestry of African Americans, Latinos, and European Americans Across the United States," *American Journal of Human Genetics* 96 (2015): 37–53.

27. A. Vander et al., *Human Physiology: The Mechanisms of Body Function*, 8th ed. (McGraw-Hill, 2001).

28. F. Xu et al., "The Roles of Epigenetics Regulation in Bone Metabolism and Osteoporosis," *Frontiers in Cell and Developmental Biology* 8 (2021): 619301.

29. T. Demeke et al., "Lower Bone Mineral Density in Somali Women Living in Sweden Compared with African-Americans," *Archives of Osteoporosis* 10, no. 1 (2015): 208; R.

Heffron et al., "Bone Mineral Density, Nutrient Intake, and Physical Activity Among Young Women from Uganda," *Archives of Osteoporosis* 17, no. 1 (2022): 134.

30. M. Anderson, *A Rising Share of the U.S. Black Population Is Foreign Born.*
31. Leslie and ASBMR Task Force on Clinical Algorithms for Fracture Risk, "Effect of Race/Ethnicity on United States FRAX Calculations."
32. A. S. Levey et al., "A New Equation to Estimate Glomerular Filtration Rate," *Annals of Internal Medicine* 150, no. 9 (2009): 604–12; erratum in *Annals of Internal Medicine* 155, no. 6 (2011): 408.
33. N. D. Eneanya et al., "Reconsidering the Consequences of Using Race to Estimate Kidney Function," *Journal of the American Medical Association* 32, no. 2 (2019): 113–14.
34. M. A. Bredella, "Sex Differences in Body Composition," *Advances in Experimental Medicine and Biology* 1043 (2017): 9–27.
35. R. Milić et al., "Serum Creatinine Concentrations in Male and Female Elite Swimmers. Correlation with Body Mass Index and Evaluation of Estimated Glomerular Filtration Rate," *Clinical Chemistry and Laboratory Medicine* 49, no. 2 (2011): 285–89.
36. J. Hsu, et al., "Higher Serum Creatinine Concentrations in Black Patients with Chronic Kidney Disease: Beyond Nutritional Status and Body Composition," *Clinical Journal of the American Society of Nephrology* 3, no. 4 (2008): 992–97; D. A. Vyas et al., "Hidden in Plain Sight—Reconsidering the Use of Race Correction in Clinical Algorithms," *New England Journal of Medicine* 383, no. 9 (2020): 874–82.
37. Eneanya et al., "Reconsidering the Consequences."
38. Vyas et al., "Hidden in Plain Sight."
39. M. Raynaud et al., "Race-Free Estimated Glomerular Filtration Rate Equation in Kidney Transplant Recipients: Development and Validation Study," *British Medical Journal* 381 (2023): e073654.
40. P. Jamshidi et al., "Investigating Associated Factors with Glomerular Filtration Rate: Structural Equation Modeling," *BMC Nephrology* 21, no. 1 (2020): 30.
41. J. A. Diao et al., "Implications of Race Adjustment in Lung-Function Equations," *New England Journal of Medicine* 390, no. 22 (2024): 2083–97.
42. V. Nauman, "Tackling Discrimination in the NFL: How the Recent CTE Race-Norming Agreement Highlights the Need to Provide Broader Anti-discrimination Protections for NFL Players Through Collective Bargaining Agreements," *William & Mary Business Law Review* 14, no. 2 (2023): 489.
43. K. Henry and N. Davenport v. National Football League and NFL Properties, LLC, No. 2:20-cv-04165 (E. D. Pa., August 25, 2020), complaint at 1–5.
44. T. McGrath et al., "Acquisition of Chess Knowledge in AlphaZero," *Proceedings of the National Academy of Sciences of the United States of America* 119, no. 47 (2022): e2206625119.
45. R. Poplin et al., "Prediction of Cardiovascular Risk Factors from Retinal Fundus Photographs Via Deep Learning," *Nature Biomedical Engineering* 2, no. 3 (2018): 158–64.
46. L. Seyyed-Kalantari et al., "Underdiagnosis Bias of Artificial Intelligence Algorithms Applied to Chest Radiographs in Under-Served Patient Populations," *Nature Medicine* 27, no. 12 (2021): 2176–82.
47. J. W. Gichoya et al., "AI Recognition of Patient Race in Medical Imaging: A Modelling Study," *Lancet Digital Health* 4, no. 6 (2022): e406–14.
48. Y. Yang et al., "The Limits of Fair Medical Imaging AI in Real-World Generalization," *Nature Medicine* 30, no. 10 (2024): 2838–48.

49. "Artificial Intelligence and Machine Learning (AI/ML)–Enabled Medical Devices," US Food and Drug Administration, March 25, 2025, https://www.fda.gov/medical -devices/software-medical-device-samd/artificial-intelligence-and-machine-learning -aiml-enabled-medical-devices.

50. S. A. Tishkoff et al., "The Genetic Structure and History of Africans and African Americans," *Science* 324, no. 5930 (2009): 1035–44.

51. C. H. Welsh et al., "Operation Everest. II: Spirometric and Radiographic Changes in Acclimatized Humans at Simulated High Altitudes," *American Review of Respiratory Disease* 147, no. 5 (1993): 1239–44.

52. J. A. Omiye et al., "Large Language Models Propagate Race-Based Medicine," *NPJ Digital Medicine* 6, no. 1 (2023): 195.

53. J. Gravel et al., "Learning to Fake It: Limited Responses and Fabricated References Provided by ChatGPT for Medical Questions," *Mayo Clinic Proceedings: Digital Health* 1, no. 3 (2023): 226–34.

10. PRECISION MEDICINE

1. S. F. Terry, "Obama's Precision Medicine Initiative," *Genetic Testing and Molecular Biomarkers* 19, no. 3 (2015): 113–14.

2. F. S. Collins and H. Varmus, "A New Initiative on Precision Medicine," *New England Journal of Medicine* 372, no. 9 (2015): 793–95.

3. All of Us Research Program Investigators et al., "The 'All of Us' Research Program," *New England Journal of Medicine* 381, no. 7 (2019): 668–76.

4. All of Us Research Program Division of Engagement and Outreach, *Annual Report, 2023* (National Institutes of Health, 2023), https://allofus.nih.gov/sites/default/files /508%20Compliant_AoU_Division%20of%20Engagement%20%26%20Outreach%20 Annual%20Repot_Final.pdf.

5. "All of Us Research Program Establishes New Center for Linkage and Acquisition of Data," National Institutes of Health, October 12, 2023, https://allofus.nih.gov/news -events/announcements/all-us-research-program-establishes-new-center-linkage-and -acquisition-data.

6. N. Krieger, *Epidemiology and the People's Health: Theory and Context*, 2nd ed. (Oxford University Press, 2024); A. Geronimus, *Weathering: The Extraordinary Stress of Ordinary Life in an Unjust Society* (Little, Brown, Spark, 2023); J. L. Graves and A. Goodman, *Racism, Not Race: Answers to Frequently Asked Questions* (Columbia University Press, 2022).

7. See, for example, the categories used in All of Us Research Program Genomics Investigators, "Genomic Data in the All of Us Research Program," *Nature* 627, no. 8003 (2024): 340–46.

8. National Academies of Sciences, Engineering, and Medicine, *Using Population Descriptors in Genetics and Genomics Research: A New Framework for an Evolving Field* (National Academies Press, 2023).

9. M. N. Pelter and R. S. Druz, "Precision Medicine: Hype or Hope?," *Trends in Cardiovascular Medicine* 34, no. 2 (2024): 120–25.

10. S. Stearns and R. Medzhitov, *Evolutionary Medicine* (Sinauer, 2016).

11. M. E. Franks et al., "Thalidomide," *Lancet* 363, no. 9423 (2004): 1802–11.

12. G. R. Venning, "Identification of Adverse Reactions to New Drugs. IV—Verification of Suspected Adverse Reactions," *British Medical Journal (Clinical Research Edition)* 286, no. 6364 (1983): 544–47.

13. D. K. Wysowski and L. Swartz, "Adverse Drug Event Surveillance and Drug Withdrawals in the United States, 1969–2002: The Importance of Reporting Suspected Reactions," *Archives of Internal Medicine* 165, no. 12 (2005): 1363–69.

14. L. E. Russell et al., "Pharmacogenomics in the Era of Next Generation Sequencing—From Byte to Bedside," *Drug Metabolism Reviews* 53, no. 2 (2021): 253–78.

15. Stearns and Medzhitov, *Evolutionary Medicine.*

16. Russell et al., "Pharmacogenomics."

17. V. M. Lauschke and M. Ingelman-Sundberg, "Prediction of Drug Response and Adverse Drug Reactions: From Twin Studies to Next Generation Sequencing," *European Journal of Pharmaceutical Sciences* 130 (2019): 65–77.

18. Y. Gasche et al., "Codeine Intoxication Associated with Ultrarapid CYP2D6 Metabolism," *New England Journal of Medicine* 351, no. 27 (2004): 2827–31 (erratum in *New England Journal of Medicine* 352, no. 6 [2005]: 638); G. P. Aithal et al., "Association of Polymorphisms in the Cytochrome P450 CYP2C9 with Warfarin Dose Requirement and Risk of Bleeding Complications," *Lancet* 353, no. 9154 (1999): 717–19; A. R. Shuldiner et al., "Association of Cytochrome P450 2C19 Genotype with the Antiplatelet Effect and Clinical Efficacy of Clopidogrel Therapy," *Journal of the American Medical Association* 302, no. 8 (2009): 849–57.

19. A. B. van Kuilenburg et al., "Clinical Implications of Dihydropyrimidine Dehydrogenase (DPD) Deficiency in Patients with Severe 5-Fluorouracil-Associated Toxicity: Identification of New Mutations in the DPD Gene," *Clinical Cancer Research* 6, no. 12 (2000): 4705–12.

20. G. Plopper et al., eds., *Lewin's Cells*, 3rd ed. (Jones & Bartlett Learning, 2015).

21. C. Yan et al., "Impact of Germline and Somatic Missense Variations on Drug Binding Sites," *Pharmacogenomics Journal* 17, no. 2 (2017): 128–36.

22. M. Lek et al., "Analysis of Protein-Coding Genetic Variation in 60,706 Humans," *Nature* 536, no. 7616 (2016): 285–91.

23. Y. Zhou et al., "Rare Genetic Variability in Human Drug Target Genes Modulates Drug Response and Can Guide Precision Medicine," *Scientific Advances* 7, no. 36 (2021): eabi6856.

24. See Graves and Goodman, *Racism, Not Race*, chap. 2.

25. T. Shiina et al., "The HLA Genomic Loci Map: Expression, Interaction, Diversity and Disease," *Journal of Human Genetics* 54, no. 1 (2009): 15–39.

26. Lauschke and Ingelman-Sundberg, "Prediction of Drug Response."

27. Russell et al., "Pharmacogenomics in the Era of Next Generation Sequencing."

28. K. Maekawa et al., "Development of a Simple Genotyping Method for the HLA-A*31:01-Tagging SNP in Japanese," *Pharmacogenomics* 16, no. 15 (2015): 1689–99.

29. Russell et al., "Pharmacogenomics in the Era of Next Generation Sequencing."

30. R. Khosravan et al., "Population Pharmacokinetic/Pharmacodynamic Modeling of Sunitinib by Dosing Schedule in Patients with Advanced Renal Cell Carcinoma or Gastrointestinal Stromal Tumor," *Clinical Pharmacokinetics* 55, no. 10 (2016): 1251–69.

31. M. Robson et al., "Olaparib for Metastatic Breast Cancer in Patients with a Germline BRCA Mutation," *New England Journal of Medicine* 377, no. 6 (2017): 523–33.

32. R. Huddart et al., "Are Randomized Controlled Trials Necessary to Establish the Value of Implementing Pharmacogenomics in the Clinic?," *Clinical Pharmacology and Therapeutics* 106, no. 2 (2019): 284–86.

33. E. Cecchin and G. Stocco, "Pharmacogenomics and Personalized Medicine," *Genes* 11, no. 6 (2020): 679; D. R. Camidge et al., "Race and Ethnicity Representation in Clinical Trials: Findings from a Literature Review of Phase I Oncology Trials," *Future Oncology* 17, no. 24 (2021): 3271–80; Russell et al., "Pharmacogenomics in the Era of Next Generation Sequencing"; E. F. Magavern et al., "Health Equality, Race and Pharmacogenomics," *British Journal of Clinical Pharmacology* 88, no. 1 (2022): 27–33.

34. Camidge et al., "Race and Ethnicity Representation."

35. Magavern et al., "Health Equality, Race and Pharmacogenomics."

36. H3Africa Consortium et al., "Enabling the Genomic Revolution in Africa," *Science* 344, no. 6190 (2014): 1346–48; A. Matimba et al., "Is There a Role of Pharmacogenomics in Africa," *Global Health, Epidemiology and Genomics* 1 (2016): e9.

37. S. E. Kimmel et al., "A Pharmacogenetic Versus a Clinical Algorithm for Warfarin Dosing," *New England Journal of Medicine* 369, no. 24 (2013): 2283–93.

38. Magavern et al., "Health Equality, Race and Pharmacogenomics."

39. B. Cross et al., "Being Precise with Anticoagulation to Reduce Adverse Drug Reactions: Are We There Yet?," *Pharmacogenomics Journal* 24, no. 2 (2024): 7.

40. M. G. Naranjo et al., "Interethnic Variability in CYP2D6, CYP2C9, and CYP2C19 Genes and Predicted Drug Metabolism Phenotypes Among 6060 Ibero- and Native Americans: RIBEF-CEIBA Consortium Report on Population Pharmacogenomics," *Omics* 22, no. 9 (2018): 575–88.

41. C. Céspedes-Garro et al., "Worldwide Interethnic Variability and Geographical Distribution of CYP2C9 Genotypes and Phenotypes," *Expert Opinion on Drug Metabolism & Toxicology* 11, no. 12 (2015): 1893–905; Cross et al., "Being Precise."

42. K. D. Christensen et al., "Assessing the Costs and Cost-Effectiveness of Genomic Sequencing," *Journal of Personalized Medicine* 5, no. 4 (2015): 470–86.

43. H. V. Fineberg, "A Successful and Sustainable Health System—How to Get There from Here," *New England Journal of Medicine* 366 (2012): 1020–27.

44. M. Verbelen et al., "Cost-Effectiveness of Pharmacogenetic-Guided Treatment: Are We There Yet?," *Pharmacogenomics Journal* 17, no. 5 (2017): 395–402.

45. Verbelen et al., "Cost-Effectiveness of Pharmacogenetic-Guided Treatment."

46. S. A. Morris et al., "Cost Effectiveness of Pharmacogenetic Testing for Drugs with Clinical Pharmacogenetics Implementation Consortium (CPIC) Guidelines: A Systematic Review," *Clinical Pharmacology and Therapeutics* 112, no. 6 (2022): 1318–28.

47. T. Morrow and L. H. Felcone, "Defining the Difference: What Makes Biologics Unique," *Biotechnology Healthcare* 1, no. 4 (2004): 24–29.

48. A. Lange et al., "A Systematic Review of Cost-Effectiveness of Monoclonal Antibodies for Metastatic Colorectal Cancer," *European Journal of Cancer* 50, no. 1 (2014): 40–49.

49. F. De Majo and L. J. De Windt, "RNA Therapeutics for Heart Disease," *Biochemical Pharmacology* 155 (2018): 468–78.

50. M. A. Chisholm-Burns et al., "Evaluation of Racial and Socioeconomic Disparities in Medication Pricing and Pharmacy Access and Services," *American Journal of Health-System Pharmacy* 74, no. 10 (2017): 653–68.

51. "How do I find the best severe combined immunodeficiency (SCID) doctor near me?," MediFind, accessed July 12, 2024, https://www.medifind.com/conditions/severe-combined-immunodeficiency-scid/4800/doctors?page=1.

52. S. Lindeberg, *Food and Western Disease: Health and Nutrition From an Evolutionary Perspective*, (Wiley-Blackwell, 2016); R. Nesse, *Good Reasons for Bad Feelings: Insights From the Frontier of Evolutionary Psychiatry*, (Dutton, 2019).

53. P. D. Darbre, "Endocrine Disruptors and Obesity," *Current Obesity Reports* 6, no. 1 (2017): 18–27; A. Gupta et al., "Brain–Gut–Microbiome Interactions in Obesity and Food Addiction," *Nature Reviews Gastroenterology & Hepatology* 17, no. 11 (2020): 655–72; N. Panera et al., "Genetics, Epigenetics and Transgenerational Transmission of Obesity in Children," *Frontiers in Endocrinology* 13 (2022): 1006008; B. Masood and M. Moorthy, "Causes of Obesity: A Review," *Clinical Medicine* 23, no. 4 (2023): 284–91.

54. Panera et al., "Genetics, Epigenetics."

55. V. Kumar, A. Abbas, J. Aster, A. Deyrup, and A. Das, *Robbins & Kumar Basic Pathology*, 11th ed. (Elsevier, 2023).

56. B. D. Smedley et al., eds., *Unequal Treatment: Confronting Racial and Ethnic Disparities in Health Care* (National Academies Press, 2002).

57. K. Fiscella and M. R. Sanders, "Racial and Ethnic Disparities in the Quality of Health Care," *Annual Review of Public Health* 37 (2016): 375–94.

58. J. E. Dalen et al., "Why Do So Many Americans Oppose the Affordable Care Act?," *American Journal of Medicine* 128, no. 8 (2015): 807–10.

59. Fiscella and Sanders, "Racial and Ethnic Disparities."

60. Dalen et al., "Why Do So Many Americans Oppose the Affordable Care Act?"

61. M. Kozlov and R. Ryan, "How Trump 2.0 Is Slashing NIH Backed Research—In Charts," *Nature News*, April 10, 2025, https://www.nature.com/articles/d41586-025-01099-8.

62. J. Stein and J. Bogage, "Trump Plans to Claim Sweeping Powers to Cancel Federal Spending," *Washington Post*, June 7, 2024, https://www.washingtonpost.com/business/2024/06/07/trump-budget-impoundment-congress/.

63. N. Kapucu and D. Moynihan, "Trump's (Mis)management of the COVID-19 Pandemic in the US," *Policy Studies* 42, nos. 5–6 (2021): 592–610.

11. DOING THE WORK TO CHANGE MEDICAL MINDS

1. J. L. Graves, *The Emperor's New Clothes: Biological Theories of Race at the Millennium* (Rutgers University Press, 2001); J. L. Graves, *The Race Myth: Why We Pretend Race Exists in America* (Dutton, 2004).

2. H. S. Meyer et al., "Biology and Race: *The Emperor's New Clothes: Biological Theories of Race at the Millennium*," *Journal of the American Medical Association* 287, no. 1 (2002): 115–16.

3. J. Botta, "Shaking a Shared Delusion: Andrea Deyrup Combats Race-Based Medicine," Duke University School of Medicine, February 8, 2023, https://medschool.duke.edu/stories/shaking-shared-delusion-andrea-deyrup-combats-race-based-medicine.

4. J. Bauml et al., "Frequency of EGFR and KRAS Mutations in Patients with Non Small Cell Lung Cancer by Racial Background: Do Disparities Exist?," *Lung Cancer* 81, no. 3 (2013): 347–53.

5. R. Dennison et al., "Lyme Disease with Erythema Migrans and Seventh Nerve Palsy in an African-American Man," *Cureus* 11, no. 12 (2019): e6509.

6. A. Rana et al., "Representation of Skin Colors in Images of Patients with Lupus," *Arthritis Care & Research* 74, no. 11 (2022): 1835–41.

7. "Complete Anatomy 2023: Now with Model Customization," Complete Anatomy Community Blog, November 14, 2022, https://3d4medical.com/blog/complete-anatomy-2023-update.

8. Z. Qureshi and M. Suleman, *Anti-Racist Medicine* (Elsevier, 2025).

9. M. K. Evans et al., "Race in Medicine—Genetic Variation, Social Categories, and Paths to Health Equity," *New England Journal of Medicine* 385, no. 14 (2021): e45.

10. See, for example, S. A. Tishkoff et al., "The Genetic Structure and History of Africans and African Americans," *Science* 324, no. 5930 (2009): 1035–44.

11. A. Deyrup and J. L. Graves Jr., "Racial Biology and Medical Misconceptions," *New England Journal of Medicine* 386, no. 6 (2022): 501–3.

12. A. Deyrup, "Pathology Central Race in Medicine: Keloids," posted October 28, 2021, YouTube, https://www.youtube.com/watch?v=cnNP_X5Hf70&t=2s.

13. See, for example, T. Tulandi et al., "Prospective Study of Intraabdominal Adhesions Among Women of Different Races with or Without Keloids," *American Journal of Obstetrics and Gynecology* 204, no. 2 (2011): 132.e1–4; W. G. Young et al., "Incidence of Keloid and Risk Factors Following Head and Neck Surgery," *JAMA Facial Plastic Surgery* 16, no. 5 (2014): 379–80.

14. A. Li et al., "Race in the Reading: A Study of Problematic Uses of Race and Ethnicity in a Prominent Pediatrics Textbook," *Academic Medicine* 97, no. 10 (2022): 1521–27.

15. T. K. McInerny et al., *American Academy of Pediatrics Textbook of Pediatric Care*, 2nd ed. (AAP, 2016).

16. S. R. Johnson, "American Academy of Pediatrics Moves to Erase 'Race-Based Medicine,'" *US News & World Report*, May 2, 2022, https://www.usnews.com/news/health-news/articles/2022-05-02/american-academy-of-pediatrics-moves-to-erase-race-based-medicine; J. L. Wright et al., "Eliminating Race-Based Medicine," *Pediatrics* 150, no. 1 (2022): e2022057998.

17. F. Pratto et al., "Social Dominance Orientation: A Personality Variable Predicting Social and Political Attitudes," *Journal of Personality and Social Psychology* 67 (1994): 741–63.

18. B. Lepièce et al., "Social Dominance Theory and Medical Specialty Choice," *Advances in Health Sciences Education: Theory and Practice* 21, no. 1 (2016): 79–92.

19. S. Heiser, "Press Release: The Majority of U.S. Medical Students Are Women, New Data Show," Association of American Medical Colleges, December 9, 2019, https://www.aamc.org/news/press-releases/majority-us-medical-students-are-women-new-data-show.

20. C. J. Bowen et al., "Medical School Research Ranking Is Associated with Gender Inequality in MSTP Application Rates," *BMC Medical Education* 18, no. 1 (2018): 187.

21. One of the early iterations of this lecture can be viewed at https://www.youtube.com/watch?v=V525mqBj8uA.

22. J. L. Graves Jr., "The Myth of the Genetically Sick African," *Genealogy* 6, no. 1 (2022): 15; P. Henry et al., "Embedded Racism: Inequitable Niche Construction as a Neglected Evolutionary Process Affecting Health," *Evolution, Medicine, and Public Health* 11, no. 1 (2023): 112–25.

23. D. Tweedy, *Black Man in a White Coat: A Doctor's Reflections on Race and Medicine* (Picador, 2016).

24. E. T. Norris et al., "Genetic Ancestry, Admixture and Health Determinants in Latin America," *BMC Genomics* 19, no. S8 (2018): 861.

25. A. B. Conley et al., "A Comparative Analysis of Genetic Ancestry and Admixture in the Colombian Populations of Chocó and Medellín," *G3* 7, no. 10 (2017): 3435–47.

26. National Academies of Sciences, Engineering, and Medicine, *Using Population Descriptors in Genetics and Genomics Research: A New Framework for an Evolving Field* (National Academies Press, 2023).

27. "2024 Annual Meeting Schedule: Bringing Education to Life," United States and Canadian Academy of Pathology, March 23–28, 2024, https://2024am.uscap.org/schedule/.

28. "Active Physicians Who Identified as Black or African American," American Association of Medical Colleges, accessed June 23, 2024, https://www.aamc.org/data-reports/workforce/data/active-physicians-black-african-american-2021.

29. J. W. Jacobs et al., "Analysis of Race and Ethnicity Among United States Medical Board Leadership," *Journal of Women's Health* 32, no. 9 (2023): 921–26.

30. A. J. Hill et al., "Physician-Patient Race-Match Reduces Patient Mortality," *Journal of Health Economics* 92 (2023): 102821.

31. STAT News, "Med Schools See Steep Drop in Enrollment of Black and Hispanic Students After SCOTUS Ruling," Health Leaders, January 10, 2025, https://www.healthleadersmedia.com/cmo/med-schools-see-steep-drop-enrollment-black-and-hispanic-students-after-scotus-ruling.

32. J. L. Graves and A. Goodman, *Racism, Not Race: Answers to Frequently Asked Questions* (Columbia University Press, 2022).

33. J. L. Graves, "Science, Empire, and US Imperialism," in *The Routledge History of American Science*, ed. T. Kneeland (Routledge, 2022), 231–42.

34. J. Hochschild and M. Sen, "American's Attitudes on Individual or Racially Reflected Genetic Inheritance," in *Reconsidering Race: Social Science Perspectives on Racial Categories in the Age of Genomics*, ed. K. Suzuki and D. A. Von Vacano (Oxford University Press, 2018: 32–49); J. L. Graves, "Out of Africa: Where Faith, Race, and Science Collide," in *Critical Approaches to Science and Religion*, ed. M. Sheldon et al. (Columbia University Press, 2023: 255–76); S. Outram et al., "Genes, Race, and Causation: US Public Perspectives About Racial Difference," *Race and Social Problems* 10 (2018): 79–90.

35. J. L. Graves, "Why We Must Teach Our Students About Race," *American Biology Teacher* 85, no. 3 (2023): 133; J. L. Graves, "Why We Should Teach Our Students About Race," *Reports of the National Center for Science Education* 22, no. 3 (2002): 23–26.

36. M. Berkman and E. Plutzer, *Evolution, Creationism, and the Battle to Control America's Classrooms* (Cambridge University Press, 2010).

37. See the National Center for Science Education website: https://ncse.ngo/.

38. G. Branch et al., "Teaching Evolution in U.S. Public Middle Schools: Results of the First National Survey," *Evolution: Education and Outreach* 14, no. 8 (2021); L. S. Mead and A. Mates, "Why Science Standards Are Important to a Strong Science Curriculum and How States Measure Up," *Evolution: Education and Outreach* 2 (2009): 359–71; "Teaching Evolution: Do State Science Standards Matter?," *Reports of the National Center for Science Education* 21, nos. 1–2 (2001).

39. Q. Scanlan and M. Osborne, "Donald Trump Returns to Stage with Speech at North Carolina GOP Convention," ABC News, June 5, 2021, https://abcnews.go.com/Politics/donald-trump-returns-stage-speech-north-carolina-gop/story?id=78107039.

40. "Donald Trump Speech Transcript at North Carolina GOP Convention Dinner June 5," Rev, June 5, 2021, https://www.rev.com/blog/transcripts/donald-trump-speech-transcript-at-north-carolina-gop-convention-dinner-june-5.

41. C. Stout and T. Wilburn, "CRT Map: Efforts to Restrict Teaching About Racism and Bias Have Multiplied Across the U.S.," Chalkbeat, July 22, 2021, https://www.chalkbeat.org/22525983/map-critical-race-theory-legislation-teaching-racism.

42. K. Managan, "'A Slap in the Face': How UT-Austin Axed a DEI Division," *Chronicle of Higher Education*, June 27, 2024.

43. B. M. Donovan et al., "How Can We Make Genetics Education More Humane?," in *Contributions from Biology Education Research*, ed. M. Haskel-Ittah and A. Yarden (Springer, 2021); B. M. Donovan et al., "From Basic to Humane Genomics Literacy: How Different Types of Genetics Curricula Could Influence Anti-essentialist Understandings of Race," *Science & Education* 29, no. 6 (2020), 1479–1511; B. M. Donovan et al., "Toward a More Humane Genetics Education: Learning About the Social and Quantitative Complexities of Human Genetic Variation Research Could Reduce Racial Bias in Adolescent and Adult Populations," *Science Education* 103, no. 3 (2019): 529–60.

44. Graves and Goodman, *Racism, Not Race*.

45. C. R. Lucey and A. Saguil, "The Consequences of Structural Racism on MCAT Scores and Medical School Admissions: The Past Is Prologue," *Academic Medicine* 95, no. 3 (2020): 351–56.

46. K. Ripp and L. Braun, "Race/Ethnicity in Medical Education: An Analysis of a Question Bank for Step 1 of the United States Medical Licensing Examination," *Teaching and Learning in Medicine* 29, no. 2 (2017): 115–22.

47. "Press Release: Murphy Introduces Bill to Ban DEI in Medicine," U.S. Congressman Gregory F. Murphy, M.D., March 19, 2024, https://murphy.house.gov/media/press-releases/murphy-introduces-bill-ban-dei-medicine.

48. J. L. Graves et al., "Historically Black Colleges and Universities Have Affirmative Action Solutions. But They Need Help," *Scientific American*, July 18, 2023, https://www.scientificamerican.com/article/historically-black-colleges-and-universities-have-affirmative-action-solutions-but-they-need-help/.

49. A. Figueroa, "States Urged by Biden Administration to Rectify Underfunding of the Land-Grant HBCUs," NC Newsline, September 19, 2023, https://ncnewsline.com/2023/09/19/states-urged-by-biden-administration-to-rectify-underfunding-of-land-grant-hbcus/.

50. A. Harris, *The State Must Provide: Why America's Colleges Have Always Been Unequal and How to Set Them Right* (Ecco, 2021).

51. Figueroa, "States Urged."

CONCLUSION: BUILDING A WORLD WHERE WE CAN ALL LIVE WELL

1. J. L. Graves, "Out of Africa: Where Faith, Race, and Science Collide," in *Critical Approaches to Science and Religion*, ed. M. Sheldon et al. (Columbia University Press, 2023: 255–76).

2. T. Dobzhansky, "Nothing in Biology Makes Sense Except in the Light of Evolution," *American Biology Teacher* 35, no. 3 (1973): 125–29.

3. R. Nesse and G. C. Williams, *Why We Get Sick: The New Science of Darwinian Medicine* (Vintage, 1994).

4. J. L. Graves et al., "Evolutionary Science as a Method to Facilitate Higher Level Thinking and Reasoning in Medical Training," *Evolution, Medicine, and Public Health* 2016, no. 1 (2016): 358–68.

5. J. L. Graves, "Evolutionary Versus Racial Medicine: Why It Matters," in *Race and the Genetic Revolution: Science, Myth and Culture*, ed. S. Krimsky and S. Sloan (Columbia University Press, 2011: 142–70).

6. P. Ivey Henry, M. Spence Beaulieu, A. Bradford, J. Graves, Embedded racism: Inequitable niche construction as a neglected evolutionary process affecting health. *Evolution, Medicine, and Public Health* 11, no. 1(2023):112–25.

7. R. S. Garcia, "The Misuse of Race in Medical Diagnosis," *Pediatrics* 113, no. 5 (2004): 1394–95; L. Szabo, "For Some Families of Color, a Painful Fight for a Cystic Fibrosis Diagnosis," *New York Times,* May 29, 2024, https://www.nytimes.com/2024/05/29/well/live/cystic-fibrosis-screening.html?unlocked_article_code=1.xE0.gfOc.ZgpGHtaYZldz&smid=url-share.

8. K. E. Lohmueller et al., "Proportionally More Deleterious Genetic Variation in European than in African Populations," *Nature* 451, no. 7181 (2008): 994–97.

9. All of Us Research Program Genomics Investigators, "Genomic Data in the All of Us Research Program," *Nature* 627, no. 8003 (2024): 340–46.

10. J. L. Graves and M. R. Rose, "Against Racial Medicine," *Patterns of Prejudice* 40, nos. 4–5 (2006): 481–93; J. L. Graves, "Scylla and Charybdis: Adaptationism, Reductionism, and the Fallacy of Associating Race with Disease," in *Medical Genetics: Mutating Concepts and Evolving Disciplines,* ed. R. Ankeny and L. Parker (Kluwer Academic, 2002: 127–42); J. L. Graves, *The Emperor's New Clothes: Biological Theories of Race at the Millennium* (Rutgers University Press, 2001).

11. P. Braveman and L. Gottlieb, "The Social Determinants of Health: It's Time to Consider the Causes of the Causes," *Public Health Reports* 129, no. S2 (2014): 19–31; R. Chetty et al., "The Association Between Income and Life Expectancy in the United States, 2001–2014," *Journal of the American Medical Association* 315, no. 16 (2016): 1750–66 (erratum in *Journal of the American Medical Association* 317, no. 1 [2017]: 90); M. D. Hayward and M. P. Farina, "Dynamic Changes in the Association Between Education and Health in the United States," *Milbank Quarterly* 101, no. S1 (2023): 396–418.

12. J. L. Graves, "The Biosciences and Neo-racism," in *The Handbook of Cultural Security,* ed. Y. Watanabe (Edward Elgar, 2018: 50–71).

13. J. L. Graves and A. Goodman, *Racism, Not Race: Answers to Frequently Asked Questions* (Columbia University Press, 2022), chap. 11.

14. N. Gaber et al., "The Devil They Knew: Chemical Documents Analysis of Industry Influence on PFAS Science," *Annals of Global Health* 89, no. 1 (2023): 37; K. Steenland and A. Winquist, "PFAS and Cancer, a Scoping Review of the Epidemiologic Evidence," *Environmental Research* 194 (2021): 110690.

15. E. Schlosser, *Fast Food Empire: The Dark Side of the All-American Meal* (Mariner, 2012).

16. Henry et al., *Embedded Racism,*

17. P. McKee et al., "Malt Liquor Marketing in Inner Cities: The Role of Neighborhood Racial Composition," *Journal of Ethnicity in Substance Abuse* 10, no. 1 (2011): 24–38.

18. M. Agar and H. S. Reisinger, "A Heroin Epidemic at the Intersection of Histories: The 1960s Epidemic Among African Americans in Baltimore," *Medical Anthropology* 21, no. 2 (2002): 115–56; D. Matuskey et al., "A Preliminary Study of Dopamine D2/3 Receptor Availability and Social Status in Healthy and Cocaine Dependent Humans Imaged with [(11)C](+)PHNO," *Drug and Alcohol Dependence* 154 (2015): 167–73; R. W. Gould et al., "Social Status in Monkeys: Effects of Social Confrontation on Brain Function and Cocaine Self-Administration," *Neuropsychopharmacology* 42, no. 5 (2017): 1093–102.

19. See, for example, B. Macy, *Dopesick: Dealers, Doctors, and the Drug Company That Addicted America* (Little, Brown, 2019); J. Metzel, *Dying of Whiteness: How the Politics of Racial Resentment Is Killing America's Heartland* (Basic Books, 2018).

20. A. Lee et al., "Social and Environmental Factors Influencing Obesity," in *Endotext* [Internet], ed. K. R. Feingold et al. (MDText.com, 2019), https://www.endotext.org/.

21. W. Jefferson et al., *African Americans and Climate Change: An Unequal Burden* (Congressional Black Caucus Foundation, 2004), http://sustainablecommunitydevelopmentgroup .org/wordpress/wp-content/uploads/2013/06/African-Americans-Climate-Report -l.pdf.

22. M. Scheifstein, "Study of Hurricane Katrina's Dead Show Most Were Old, Lived Near Levee Breaches," *Times-Picayune*, August 28, 2009, https://www.nola.com/news/weather /study-of-hurricane-katrinas-dead-show-most-were-old-lived-near-levee-breaches /article_35741734-68e1-575e-86d0-29366eed38e5.html.

23. M. A. Bender et al., "Modeled Impact of Anthropogenic Warming on the Frequency of Intense Atlantic Hurricanes," *Science* 327, no. 5964 (2010): 454–58; T. Knutson, "Global Warming and Hurricanes," Geodynamics Fluid Laboratory, accessed July 16, 2024, https://www.gfdl.noaa.gov/global-warming-and-hurricanes/.

24. "NASA Finds Summer 2024 Hottest to Date," NASA, September 11, 2024, https://www .nasa.gov/earth/nasa-finds-summer-2024-hottest-to-date/.

25. G. Carlson, *Human Health and the Climate Crisis* (Jones & Bartlett Learning, 2023).

26. "Locally Acquired Malaria Cases Identified in the United States," CDC Emergency Preparedness and Response, June 26, 2023, https://emergency.cdc.gov/han/2023/han00494 .asp.

27. J. D. Mayer, *Running on Race: Racial Politics in Presidential Campaigns 1960–2000* (Random House, 2002).

28. Metzel, *Dying of Whiteness*.

29. C. Childers, "Breaking down the South's economic underperformance: Rooted in Racism and Economic Exploitation: Part Two," Economic Policy Institute, June 11, 2024, https://www.epi.org/publication/rooted-racism-part2/?mc_cid=5a981260f8&mc_eid =0c91522649.

30. W. Shirer, *The Rise and Fall of the Third Reich: A History of Nazi Germany* (Simon & Schuster, 1959).

31. A. O'Kruk and C. Merrill, "Donald Trump's Criminal Cases, in One Place," CNN Politics, January 10, 2025, https://www.cnn.com/interactive/2023/07/politics/trump-indictments -criminal-cases/.

32. Mayer, *Running on Race*.

33. G. Grossi, "FDA Quietly Removes Draft Guidance on Diversity in Clinical Trials," AJMC, January 31, 2025, https://www.ajmc.com/view/fda-quietly-removes-draft-guidance -on-diversity-in-clinical-trials-following-executive-order-on-dei.

34. *Guidance on HIV Prevention and Pre-exposure Prophylaxis (PrEP)* (Centers for Disease Control and Prevention, 2017), https://www.cdc.gov/hiv/pdf/risk/prep/cdc-hiv-prep -guidelines-2017.pdf (page no longer available).

35. Shirer, *The Rise and Fall of the Third Reich*.

36. M. Mason, "Republicans Blame DEI for the LA Fires. This Fire Captain Disagrees," *Politico*, January 15, 2025, https://www.politico.com/news/2025/01/15/republicans-dei -la-fires-00198551; D. E. Sanger, "Trump Blames D.E.I. and Biden for Crash Under His Watch," *New York Times*, February 1, 2025, https://www.nytimes.com/2025/01/30/us /politics/trump-plane-crash-dei-faa-diversity.html.

37. C. Megarian, "Trump Orders Temporary Funding Freeze That Could Affect Trillions of Dollars," Associated Press, January 28, 2025, https://www.pbs.org/newshour/politics /trump-orders-temporary-funding-freeze-that-could-affect-trillions-of-dollars.

38. L. Martin, "Bureau Clergyman: How the FBI Colluded with an African American Televangelist to Destroy Dr. Martin Luther King, Jr.," *Religion and American Culture: A Journal of Interpretation* 28, no. 1 (2018): 1–51.

39. A. Harris, *The State Must Provide: The Definitive History of Racial Inequality in American Higher Education* (Ecco, 2021).

40. C. Hiar, "Science Funding Agency Threatened with Mass Layoffs," *Politico*, February 4, 2025, https://www.politico.com/news/2025/02/04/science-funding-agency-layoffs-threat-00202426.

41. R. F. Kennedy Jr., *A Letter to Liberals: Censorship and COVID—An Attack on Science and American Ideals* (Sky Horse, Children's Health Defense, 2022).

42. "Vaccines and Autism," Centers for Disease Control and Prevention, accessed February 5, 2025, https://www.cdc.gov/vaccine-safety/about/autism.html.

43. W. Stone, "Senator Calls RFK Jr's Position on Race and Vaccines Dangerous," NPR, January 30, 2025, https://www.npr.org/sections/shots-health-news/2025/01/30/nx-s1-5281457/rfk-jr-vaccines-race-confirmation-hearings.

44. B. S. Hooker, "Measles-Mumps-Rubella Vaccination Timing and Autism Among Young African American Boys: A Reanalysis of CDC Data," *Translational Neurodegeneration* 3 (2014): 16; retraction in *Translational Neurodegeneration* 3 (2014): 22.

45. M. J. Maenner et al., "Prevalence and Characteristics of Autism Spectrum Disorder Among Children Aged 8 Years—Autism and Developmental Disabilities Monitoring Network, 11 Sites, United States, 2020," *Morbidity and Mortality Weekly Report Surveillance Summaries* 72, no. 2 (2023): 1–14.

46. M. Tirrell, S. Owermohle, N. Muherjee, "RFK Jr. Claims New Research Effort Will Find Cause of 'Autism Epidemic' by September," CNN Health, April 10, 2025, https://www.cnn.com/2025/04/10/health/kennedy-autism-causes/index.html.

INDEX